To Mr. Rees,

Love from

Adam   3. 10. 01

C000184283

Mary C Self.

from
MEDICINE
to
MIRACLE

from MEDICINE *to* MIRACLE

How My Faith Overcame Cancer

Dr Mary Self
and Rod Chaytor

HarperCollins*Publishers*

HarperCollins*Publishers*
77–85 Fulham Palace Road,
Hammersmith, London W6 8JB

www.**fire**and**water**.com

First published in Great Britain in 2001
by HarperCollins*Publishers*

1 3 5 7 9 10 8 6 4 2

A catalogue record for this book
is available from the British Library

ISBN 0 00 711563 6

Printed and bound in Great Britain

This book is dedicated to
Dr Robert Clewlow,
father and physician

CONTENTS

'I didn't die. I lived!
And now I'm telling the world what God did.
God tested me, He pushed me hard,
But He didn't hand me over to Death.'

Extract from Psalm 118, 'The Message' version

1

'Trust you, Little Lady, to be different!' exclaims Mr Peach. 'I wouldn't have expected anything else from a doctor's daughter, though!'

I look into the eyes of an expert. He gives me a broad smile and turns to my father who has brought me to hospital. They begin an earnest conversation in hushed tones, using unfamiliar words. I listen for a while, not wanting to be excluded. I hear snatches of words that sound important but I don't know what they mean. I do not really understand the atmosphere of alarm I have created since I told my dad about the lump on my leg.

I just feel relieved they have not mentioned the dreaded 'C' word. I push the thought from my mind. I don't know anyone young with cancer. Seventeen-year-olds don't get cancer, so I switch off and daydream. I seize the opportunity to examine the room of this kind and clever doctor whom I already hold in the greatest of awe. Tall, strong and imposing, he seems to fill the room completely and yet his manner is so gentle. I like to be called 'Little Lady'. It means he sees me as an adult. Yet underneath the surface I am as scared as only a child can be.

It is Boxing Day 1982. We are in Mr Peach's office at the Victoria Hospital, Blackpool. It is large and square with a solid desk in the centre. A grinning life-sized skeleton stands sentinel in the corner. Interesting pictures of bones and joints line the walls. I recognize some of the names from my years as a nursing cadet in the St John Ambulance Brigade and I look dreamily around as I long for the day when I, too, will have an office like this.

Mr Peach wakes me from my reverie as he approaches, swinging a small metal hammer. Instinctively, I draw back, my eyes wide with alarm. He laughingly explains: 'It's a patella hammer – to examine your knees. Hop on the couch now and let's see that leg of yours.'

Gingerly I stand and limp over to the examination area. My left knee is now so painful that my 'hop' is stiff and awkward.

Deftly, Mr Peach examines my knee. He tells me what he is doing and I feel proud when he acknowledges that I will have to learn to do this soon. He knows I want to be a doctor. I flinch as his hands encounter the lump I discovered on my leg two days before. I see a concerned look spreading over his face and my heart misses a beat. Why is everybody so twitched about this thing?

'So tell me how you found this, then,' he asks me, prodding my knee.

'I went for a jog, and when I came back my leg was hurting. Then I noticed the skin was red and warm and I could feel this lump.'

'So it has never hurt you before, then?'

'Yes, maybe a couple of times over the last few months, but it has never hurt as much as this before and I only noticed the lump on Christmas Eve.'

I think back to the first time I became aware of the throbbing pain in my knee …

It was a perfect autumn day, although late in the season. The sort that stands out in the memory with all its bright colours and bonfire smells. All Saints' Day, 1 November 1982, and my younger sister Helen – known as Hellie – and I took a break from revising for our examinations. We had been working companionably at our studies, she for her O levels and me for my A levels, for many months now. We had settled into a pleasant routine of sitting together, surrounded by our books, taking turns to make each other hot drinks. We had grown very close since our older sister, Frances – who I call Franny – left for physiotherapy training college. We had earned some time off so Mum and Dad planned this half-term trip to the Lake District for a treat. We awoke with an impatience and urgency to be away from the dreaded revision, only to be told by Mum and Dad: 'We'll leave straight after Mass.'

Hellie and I looked at each other conspiratorially. She is much braver than me, so she always does the talking.

'Oh, Mum,' she moaned, 'do we have to go to Mass today?'

'Yes,' Mum replied, in her no-arguments voice. 'It's a holy day today.'

Hellie and I pulled long faces at each other before she started to dig me in the ribs, fighting for the most room at the mirror to complete her tedious make-up routine. She can be very vain and spends ages looking after her appearance. Laughing together, we set off for Mass and then to enjoy our day out.

2

We knew that trying to dodge Mass was a long shot anyway. My family are Catholics, really strict Catholics. Our lives have been punctuated by Holy Communion and confirmation services and Holy Days of Obligation for as long as I can remember. We are never allowed to miss Mass, ever. It is written in tablets of stone. We all go to the eleven o'clock service every week, no exception. Especially now that Martin, my big brother, has stopped going to church and there has been a really big deal about it. He says that there is no such thing as God and my mum is very upset about the whole thing.

I am the middle of five children born to my parents over eight years. My youngest brother, Adrian, is four years younger than I. He is very shy but a talented musician. Martin is the eldest and four years older than me. When we were children he teased us all the time and mercilessly persecuted my sisters and me by torturing our dolls and teddy bears. He is twenty-one and in his second year reading chemistry at Manchester University. Franny is two years older than me and in her second year at college. She has also caused an almighty stir in our family because she has been going to a different church. It is not Catholic, it's Anglican. My mum and dad are very upset. They do not approve of the vicar, who is called Tony, and whenever Franny comes home there are lots of rows. But I quite like Tony; he seems to help my sister a lot. She tells me her whole life has changed since she got to know Jesus. I am very close to Franny. We share a love of sport. For years now we have gone along to gymnastics lessons and walked home together after athletics practices.

Hellie, who is fifteen, is different from Franny and me. She is dark-haired, extremely attractive and very vivacious. Sometimes Franny says Hellie is the beautiful one, I am the clever one and she is the courageous one. Just now, getting over breaking up with my boyfriend, Martyn, I wish I was the beautiful one. He is a third-year sixth-form pupil so he is older than I am and I would say that he is certainly a great deal more street-wise. I was so surprised when he took an interest in me. I don't feel that good about the way I look and he is a bit of a catch. When he asked me out I couldn't believe it. At first I just wanted a boyfriend but I soon loved being with him. I think I was probably already in love with him. When he asked me to go a bit further than just kissing, I was shocked and pleased at the same time. But – and there is always the 'but' – I knew it was wrong. So that's how it finished and now, well, I miss him dreadfully. It has been a bit of a blow to my pride, so since we broke up I have been putting all my energies into entering medical school.

My dad is a general practitioner. There is a special bond between us. When I was born, he saved my life. He has told me the story many times.

'You were awkward from the very beginning,' he begins when he recounts the drama. 'Your mum went into labour unexpectedly on the ante-natal ward and then your shoulders got stuck. I was visiting and I had to deliver you – a good job, too, or you would have died.'

'What happened next?' I always ask.

'Well, you weren't breathing so I had to resuscitate you. It was the most stressful moment of my career, trying to get a tube down your tiny wind-pipe.'

'But I made it!'

'Yes, and that's why you are called Mary. I called you after the Virgin Mary, to whom I prayed while I was trying to save your life.'

My mum is also wonderful. She is everything you would want in a mother. She is gentle and loving, but she has this way about her. It is impossible to argue with Mum. She is wise and kind and everybody loves her. Sometimes my sisters and I look at her old photographs, admiring her figure and her curls. She was so beautiful, and still is. Her eyes are clear blue and honest, her smile takes over her whole face. The earliest memory I have is sitting in her laundry basket, listening to her playing the piano and singing to me. My mum is a beautiful singer and she leads the church choir. My dad adores her. She has devoted her whole life to her family and she is, as my dad frequently tells us, the heart of our home. Although we are sheltered, I know my parents love us a lot and I have never wanted for anything. Yes, I would say we are very close.

We have lived in Blackpool all our lives. We children all attended a church primary school and went on to Catholic secondary schools. I became a proud pupil of Layton Hill Girls' Convent. The downside to this has been the total absence of boys from our life. I am just not equipped to deal with a boyfriend and I blame the system for that. What do you say to a boy when you don't know anything about them? The only thing we have ever been told about sex was one lesson when Mrs Pollock drew a pretty bad picture on the blackboard. She said that it was a man's penis but really it could have been anything. I can't believe she used to be a nurse! So, as far as boys go, I am embarrassingly shy and I never know what to say to them. I guess they find me pretty boring, really.

Last year the school merged with the Catholic boys' grammar, St Joseph's, where my brother Martin used to be a pupil. Now it is called St Mary's Roman Catholic High School. Hellie and I have both become interested in the recently formed 'God Squad' at school. There has been a big religious revival. It used to be regarded as pathetic to be seen at lunchtime Mass but now it is considered fashionable. It is all very exciting and loads of girls hang out in the chapel, singing and practising new songs. Sometimes I have gone to youth meetings with the God Squad. The last one was really fabulous. There were young people from all different types of churches – not just Catholics. Somebody got up to speak and told us about how Jesus had helped them through all kinds of problems. It made me think a lot about my own faith. Then, at the end, they asked people to go forward if they wanted to know Jesus, but I was too scared. I thought I might get laughed at. So I just stayed there with the God Squad instead …

So, back to All Saints' Day and our trip to the Lake District. The golds and yellows of the autumn leaves were just about turning to a burnished copper as we trudged through the leafy lanes of Ambleside. The thrushes were devouring the bright red berries. My sister and I kicked through the fallen piles of horse chestnut and sycamore leaves, searching for conkers and helicopter seeds.

I think I looked around with a different focus that day. I could almost see the hand of a magnificent Creator all around me. The colours, sights and sounds of autumn seemed more vivid, more beautiful than ever before. Maybe to outsiders my life seemed to have everything and to be perfectly happy, but sometimes I felt an emptiness. I had heard that the love of Jesus could transform lives and turn them around – and how I wanted that to happen! I was aware of a hunger inside me, a need to link in some way with God.

I was deep in my thoughts as we passed a tiny village church, the sort that is photographed for guide books and postcards. I noticed a creaking mossy lychgate flanked by two huge yew trees. The crumbling gravestones were covered in a tangle of ivy and weeds. Here and there a couple of vases of bright dahlias cheered up the graves.

'I'll catch you up,' I shouted to my sister, and ran down the path between the headstones. Cautiously, I pushed open the heavy oak door.

The grating sound made by the rusty hinges startled the jackdaws gathered in the steeple. Inside was dark and cool; the only noise I could hear was the distant cries of the frightened birds. Slowly my eyes adjusted to the shade and I took in my surroundings. The autumn sunlight flooded in through the stained glass windows, pictures of the saints in reds and blues dappling the stone floor in many different hues. I headed towards the altar and, as I did so, a beam of sunlight streamed in through the side window and fell on the golden cross which had been arranged as the centrepiece of the sanctuary.

I knelt close by and seemed to be bathed in a warm golden glow reflected from the cross. The peace and silence of this place was almost palpable.

'Jesus, if You are real, if You are there, take my life and transform it, too. Use me, Lord, for Your service.'

I didn't really know what I meant by it. It's the kind of prayer they say at these youth meetings where everybody seems so happy and joyful. As I stood to leave, I felt a pain shoot down my leg from my knee. It was so painful that I drew my breath in sharply.

'That's strange,' I remember thinking. 'I must have strained my muscles. Too much jogging!' I limped slowly out of the church but by the time I caught up with my sister the ache had disappeared.

I visited Franny the following weekend and she invited me to accompany her to the friendly and welcoming church she had become part of. We have always been taught, at school and at church, that there is only one truth and that is Catholicism. I know really I should pray she will see the light. However, my sister used to be really unconfident and shy and now she is a mature young woman with a joyful and carefree spirit. She is so enthusiastic about Jesus and her church that I am puzzled why everyone is so perturbed by it. But that is what it's like, being a Catholic.

I had never been to a different type of church. But off we went to the evening service on Bonfire Night and, as we huddled together around a large bonfire, Pastor Tony told us we can know God through Jesus and be reborn into a new life. Suddenly it all seemed to make sense. At the end he asked those who wished to know Jesus to go forward. This time I got up straight away and Tony smiled at me warmly as I went towards him to make my prayer. I asked the Lord to forgive my past sins and to come in and be a part of my life and that was when Jesus became a real person to me. At last I had found the way to God.

But, as I stood with Tony and he prayed with me, I remember becoming aware of an intense and throbbing pain in my left knee. The pain has not really gone away since but life has been so good I have hardly noticed it. Compared to the joy of becoming a committed Christian, it seemed insignificant. I felt as if my life was complete.

After I got converted in this way, I decided to move in from the fringes and mix more with members of the God Squad. Recently my life has revolved around folk group practices, going to chapel and other Christian youth events.

There is a sense of euphoria within the God Squad. We all feel that our lives have changed radically since we came to know Jesus personally. It is all about warmth and acceptance towards each other but, outside the group, we keep very much to ourselves. All the God Squad have been spending huge amounts of time singing and praying together and hanging out in chapel. It has begun to affect our work and everything. For the first time ever, I have got behind with my essays and homework. The thing is, it is meant to be all our lives we give to Jesus, not just a part of them. A lot of the girls try really hard and compete with each other by their attendance at Mass and folk group practices. Some of them are now praying in tongues. It basically means that they speak in this funny language. I suppose it sounds like gibberish and anyone listening would think that was what it was. They say it makes you feel all warm and peaceful. In fact, some of the girls have fallen over while praying. I mean, can you imagine? If Sister Maureen came in she would have a fit! She is our headmistress, and very prim and proper.

In all honesty, I have to admit to being a little confused by the fact that being a Christian does not make life trouble-free. Although I am filled with a tremendous love for Jesus, I do feel disappointed that I have lost a boyfriend and my marks at school are suffering because of doing all this religious stuff.

Just before Christmas, I decided to be more serious about keeping my body as a 'temple of the Holy Spirit' as it tells us to do in the Bible. So I worked out a strict regime of exercise, which means jogging two or three times a day. I am dieting now and I don't eat anything unhealthy. All my breaks and lunchtimes are spent in chapel and I have friendships only within the God Squad. I go to Mass daily and I have also started reading scripture. I have not yet received the baptism of the Holy Spirit. By that I mean that I don't yet pray in tongues or fall over or anything like that. I guess it is only a matter of time. I am so excited at the prospect; then I will be able to win back my brother and sister for the Catholic Church. That will really impress the God Squad. I have read in the gospels about the apostles receiving the Holy Spirit, performing miracles and converting thousands. We heard about another God Squad which converted the whole of their school and this is our mission now. Over Christmas we set ourselves the task of trying hard to convert our friends and families.

When the holidays started I was filled with a sense of well-being and contentment. My work picked up, my body seemed healthy and strong and I had this new faith, too. Then, on Christmas Eve, I had a conversation with my older brother, Martin. As usual we were arguing about Christianity and I was trying to convert him back.

'Christianity is just a crutch for the weak,' he said disparagingly. 'And what about earthquakes and tidal waves and famine?'

I defended my corner as I have been taught in the God Squad: all things have a purpose and good comes out of anything, even bad stuff.

'I bet you wouldn't say that if it was you!'

'What do you mean?'

'If you were suffering. Say you had cancer or something. You wouldn't be so keen then.'

'Yes I would! But, anyway, that won't happen, I won't get cancer. Now I am a Christian, God will look after me. He won't let bad things happen to me.'

My brother laughed at me and walked off with that annoying 'big brother' air of superiority. Actually, I felt he had won that round. I tidied away my books, looking forward to the enjoyable Christmas break I had promised myself. But I was disturbed by my brother's comments. I pondered the whole question of suffering for a few minutes.

'No, bad things won't happen to me,' I decided. 'Not now, not ever.' And I ran out of the room, filled with joyful anticipation. I thought that this would be the best Christmas ever!

A little later, Martin sought me out. It was late and icy cold. 'Do you fancy a jog?' he asked.

We often run together when he is home from university. I think he is quite proud of the fact that he has a sister who can almost outrun him and he takes my training as seriously as his own. He knows I have a big competition ahead. I have already represented my school and now I have a trial for the town cross-country team.

I groaned at the thought of leaving the warmth of home but sprinted up the stairs two at a time to put my running gear on. We fell into step together. The only sound I could hear was the rhythmic pounding of our training shoes as the frozen grass crunched beneath our feet. My heart soon slotted into the rhythm and I felt vibrant and alive. I tingled with the exertion of exercise and the euphoria of working my muscles.

When we got home, the heat inside the house made our faces glow. I became aware of the pain in my knee again while dressing after a hot soapy bath. I ran a hand over the smooth line of my muscles. I prodded around where the pain was and noticed the skin felt different. Even after the bath, I could still feel that my left knee was hotter than the other one and it seemed swollen.

Franny was curled up on the bed reading a textbook in preparation for her physiotherapy exams.

'Franny, could you have a look at my knee?'

'Is it still hurting you?'

'Yes. I think the muscle is in spasm or something. My knee feels swollen. It feels like a lump.'

'Yes, you're right. It feels hot, too. The skin is red, look. You'd better show Dad.'

I expected him to say it was growing pains – all adults seem to use that cover-all excuse these days – but Dad spent a long time examining my leg. He even got out a tape measure and measured round my leg to see how swollen it was. He seemed distracted.

'Mmm, it is definitely inflamed,' and he checked the measurement again. 'Is it very painful?'

'Well, it does hurt. It's hurt a couple of times over the last few months but I just thought that it was too much running.'

'I see. We will need to get it checked out after Christmas,' he said quietly as he left the room.

I looked at my watch. It was almost time for Midnight Mass, the high spot of Christmas. I pushed worries about the pain in my knee to the back of my mind and concentrated on getting ready for church.

Midnight Mass is a compulsory tradition in our family. We fill an entire church bench. My brother Adrian, at the organ, struck the chord of the first carol and I heard my mother's beautiful voice leading the choir. We three sisters sat next to my dad while Martin switched off and looked bored. The church was decked festively with holly and red candles and a huge tree, the crib laid at the foot of the altar as it has been for every Christmas I can remember.

A priest led the procession into church and carefully placed the statue of the sleeping Jesus in the manger, nestling in the straw between the stone figures of Our Lady and St Joseph. The Mass was beautiful and seemed to mean so much more than it did last year. But now I know what it is all about, you see. I am expecting something more from Christmas this year. I have asked God to use me – I don't know how, but I know that He always answers our prayers. Maybe lots of people will see the truth about Jesus or something like that. So this is what I thought about during the Mass, in between stretching out my sore leg to try and get rid of the discomfort. My dad looked at me and I thought maybe he was cross at me for fidgeting, but then he whispered and asked me if I was all right. I nodded, but by the end of the service I was in a lot of pain.

Somehow, Christmas Day itself was a bit of a let-down. Franny was ill in bed with flu and my brother spent the whole day at his girlfriend's house. The rest of us had to go to Mass again while my mum cooked Christmas dinner. Mum was a bit worried about Franny being ill and upset about Martin not being home, and Dad seemed preoccupied, too. Franny made a brief appearance when we opened the presents which were piled under the tree. I felt a bit sad because there wasn't one for me from Martyn. My parents bought me a gold cross and chain. It was very pretty and delicate and I put it on straight away. 'I'll never take it off,' I told them.

I stretched out my leg again and Dad noticed.

'Is it still hurting you?' he asked.

'Yes, it's very sore tonight,' I said, as I winced in pain.

He told me that the following day, Boxing Day, he would ring Barry Peach, an old friend of his from medical school and an orthopaedic surgeon at our local hospital.

'What's an orthopaedic surgeon?'

'A specialist doctor – someone who looks after bones and joints.' I filed the information away for medical school …

Sitting here in Mr Peach's tidy office, I replay in my mind my last run with my brother. The examination has now been completed and X-rays of my knee carried out. With a theatrical gesture, Mr Peach pins the picture up on a white illuminated box fixed on the wall in front of me.

'See here, Little Lady,' Mr Peach is pointing at the box, 'this is the problem, just here.' I look at the outline of my knee joint, labelling the bones for practice. 'Patella, tibia, fibula and femur,' I whisper under my breath, and Mr Peach smiles. And I see it – a large, white, hard lump, sitting on my bone in the wrong place.

'A limpet,' I think to myself. 'It looks just like a limpet clinging to my leg.'

My mouth is suddenly dry and my palms begin to sweat. I feel hot and cold and very, very scared. My heart is pounding in my chest as if it will burst. The voices of my dad and Mr Peach seem to recede into the distance.

'O God, don't let it be cancer,' I pray, more fervently than I would have thought possible. I know beyond a shadow of doubt that the Limpet is cruel, ugly and evil.

I lean forward and peer at it harder. Maybe by looking hard enough I can wish it away. I inspect my enemy and prepare myself for the fight ahead, for a fight I know there will be. Somewhere, deep inside, I know the Limpet will change my life beyond recognition. A terrifying and unknown beast, I realize it has the power to kill me. I know what it is. It is a tumour. It is Cancer with a big C. I'm dying.

'I am too young, Limpet,' I cry inside and I see I am hopelessly ill-equipped for this battle. I am a novice, a frightened soldier facing war for the first time.

'Why? Why me? Why now?' I ask despairingly.

The Limpet remains coldly and complacently silent.

God doesn't answer me either.

2

In the distance I hear faint strains of music. I try to place the tune and recognize 'Auld Lang Syne'. I open my eyes slowly. Lying flat on my back, I see a system of pulleys and ropes above me. I make to sit up but cry out as I feel agonizing pain in my left hip. Then comes the reassuring touch of another human hand.

'It's okay, Mary, you've had your operation.' The nurse's voice echoes, sounding too loud. 'Oh, and by the way, Happy New Year.'

I am in the Victoria Hospital, Blackpool, and I have just had my biopsy operation. My Boxing Day consultation with Mr Peach was five brief days ago and the very next day he admitted me to Ward Eight. It is midnight on New Year's Eve and I am waking up after surgery. I drift back into a heavy, drugged sleep.

Later, I awake on the first morning of 1983 with no idea what lies ahead for me this year. I manage to pull myself far enough up the bed to view the contraption that I seem to be a part of. My left leg is swathed from hip to toe in a heavy layer of bandages. A tight ring, made of leather, encircles the top of my thigh and is attached to a metal frame. The frame seems to be part of the pulley and rope system and a set of heavy metal weights finishes the whole thing off. I shift my position and pain shoots through my body. I realize it comes not from my leg but from my hip which is covered in dressings and has a large tube coming out of it. As I begin to panic at my strange and new surroundings, there is a knock on the door and Mr Peach sweeps in with a broad smile on his face.

'And how is my Little Lady today, then?'

The contraption, he tells me, is called a Thomas Splint and will be with me for a while.

'The operation was bigger than I thought would be necessary. We had to cut a lot of bone marrow away under the lump. There's only a tiny wafer of bone left. That's why you need the splint.'

'So what did you fill the hole up with?'

'We packed it with bone chips from your hip.'

'Is that why my hip hurts, then?' I am piecing together this puzzle.

'Yes, that's a bone graft and I'm afraid it will be very sore.' He looks at me apologetically. 'Be brave, Little Lady!' I nod seriously, for I would do anything he tells me.

'I have some more news.' He is grave now. 'Because the bone will be so weak, you will have to use a calliper to walk.' I know what a calliper is. I have seen musty old photographs of my father wearing one after he had a leg operation as a child. My heart sinks and I try to imagine how I will manage at school and university. As if reading my thoughts, Mr Peach says I should delay my university entrance by a year because of the difficulties of getting around.

Anxiously, I ask Mr Peach how long I am going to be in my Thomas Splint.

'I'm afraid it will be quite some time. Probably six weeks at least.'

'How will I manage? It's so uncomfortable!'

'You will get used to it,' he reassures me in his kindly way, 'and we will help you all we can.'

It feels as if the bottom has dropped out of my world. I realize I will miss my mock A level examinations, maybe even my A levels themselves.

Mr Peach goes on to explain about the tubes draining my wound, the catheter in my bladder and the intravenous drip in my arm. I feel overwhelmed by my new situation but he pats my hand, inspiring me with confidence as he says: 'Just think what a better doctor you will be for this.'

'I know, I'll be the best orthopaedic surgeon ever!' I enthuse.

'Well, you will need to get some muscles then, Little Lady!' he laughs, and leaves the room that will now become my prison for the next six weeks.

Visitors arrive in droves. My mum and dad visit me often, appearing strained and worried. I reassure them by saying, 'Don't worry, I'll be fine with my calliper.' My brothers and sisters, friends and school teachers drop in, too. I am in a great deal of pain, particularly from the hip graft, and I have lost a large amount of blood so I tire very easily. The immobility and discomfort from the Thomas Splint cause me to sleep badly and I soon feel very discouraged.

My sister Franny visits and she brings me cards with scripture verses and inspirational texts. 'Why is this happening to me now?' I ask her when the pain and tiredness become too much. 'I don't know,' she replies. 'But I do know that it says in the Bible that all situations can work together for good.' She helps me find relevant and uplifting passages of scripture and they emphasize to me why I need to have a close and personal relationship with God.

The focus of my prayer is on healing. Mr Peach explains the bone tumour has been sent off for further tests. I know there is a chance that the results could show cancer but I am determined to prove the Lord in all this and I believe God can transform the Limpet into a benign and harmless lump.

So I ask for healing and I spend more and more time praying for it. I read the gospels through, concentrating on the miracles to see how they are done. I realize that having faith is an important factor. A priest visits me and prays over my leg, placing his hands where I had the operation, now a mound of thick crepe bandages.

'Lord, we believe You can heal Mary,' he prays in a quiet intense voice. 'We ask You to glorify Yourself and make Mary well.' Then he prays in the words of the Spirit – the language of tongues. I am fascinated to hear the soft, unintelligible noises and they soothe my troubled mind. I am convinced that because the Spirit of God is present our prayers will be answered.

I have made friends with the young house officer on our ward. He breezes in, always cheerful and considerate.

'How are you, Trouble?' he says in his soft Irish voice.

'Fine, Dr Murphy, fine.'

'Call me Jimmy, as you're going to be a med student.'

'Did you know God's going to heal me, Jimmy?'

'To be sure He will, but maybe it will be through modern medicine.'

'Nope!' I exclaim. 'You see, I love the Lord and He won't let me suffer! I'll walk out of this hospital on two strong legs!'

He is the first of many visitors and nurses to whom I witness in this way.

A few days after my operation, several nurses on the ward realize I am feeling lonely and isolated in my side room. Ward Eight is a female orthopaedic ward and all the patients are immobile and elderly. Although I get plenty of visitors during the evenings, my days are long and tedious. Fixed in one position in my bed, I can't go anywhere. I find it difficult to concentrate on books and I have listened and re-listened to my music tapes. Early one morning the door bursts open.

14

'Surprise!' shout three voices in unison and three young lads file into my room in wheelchairs.

'I'm Steve.'

'I'm Pete.'

'And I'm Barry.'

'Well, I'm Mary!' I reply, eagerly. 'But what are you all doing here?'

'We've come to sympathize,' says Steve. 'We all had Thomas Splints for weeks so we know how awful it can be.'

'So what did you all do to your legs, then?' I ask.

They tell their stories which are basically the same: motorbike accidents. 'Barry's was the worst,' says Steve. 'He almost lost his leg but Mr Peach saved it.' Barry smiles shyly at me. He seems the quietest of the three.

'I had my splint for twelve weeks,' he says, 'and my leg's still in a brace.' I look at his leg extended in front of him, two large pins through his bones fixed to a metal contraption. 'At least I have my leg, though.' He smiles again at me.

We swop stories and they give me hints on how to cope with my splint. The room seems very quiet and empty when they have left. I am in a great deal of pain from the hip graft and the splint becomes more and more uncomfortable. It seems that, no matter which way I move, the leather of the ring bites into my soft flesh. I ache to be outside in the bright fresh air of crisp winter days. There is a tiny window in my room, but behind me; it feels as if light and colour have disappeared from my life. However, as the days progress and friends and neighbours hear of my predicament my room begins to fill with cards and flowers.

'Just a few days more,' I think to myself, 'and my prayers will see an answer.' The biopsy results are due and I am sure that God has healed me.

The Ward Six boys visit me often now. I begin to witness to them, explaining God can change them and heal them.

'Why did God allow my bike to crash, then?' asks Peter. 'He certainly wasn't looking out for me that day.'

'And what about my short leg?' asks Barry in his soft cheerful voice. 'I will always have to wear a boot, which will make me look awful.'

It troubles me that I feel so much doubt when I look at the problems in life which really hurt. How could God allow these young boys' lives to be damaged for ever? I am told I must not doubt God and my faith will heal me. And yet peace eludes me. I feel worried and anxious, ill and tired.

January 6 is a special day in the Catholic calendar. The twelfth day of Christmas coincides with the feast of the Epiphany. Nobody visits me. The hours pass and no-one appears. I feel even lonelier when I think about everyone being busy taking down Christmas trees and packing away decorations for next year. The crib figures will be carefully placed in their straw beds and stowed away.

In the evening, Dr Jimmy comes into my room.

'Jimmy,' I ask him, 'do you think God wants to heal me?' He looks at me and I am stunned to see tears in his eyes.

'Oh, Mary,' he sighs, 'I don't know the answer to that. I wish I did.' He seems troubled, but then I know from our conversations that life as a house officer is not easy.

'So why are you here so late, Jimmy?' I continue, trying to sound cheerful.

'Well, I'm a vampire tonight,' he laughs, seeming to have recovered his usual good mood. 'I need to take your blood, Little Lady.'

'Why do you need to do that?' I know this is out of the usual routine.

'Well, tomorrow we have to take you to the operating theatre.' He pauses for a few seconds. 'To … check your dressings.'

'Do I need to go to sleep for that, then?' I ask, surprised, as the nurses have checked my dressings several times already in previous days.

'Yes, you do – it could be painful,' he replies slowly, concentrating on his task.

'So what's the transfusion for?' I ask curiously, noticing a form requesting a blood cross-match. After a moment's silence, Jimmy looks up from my arm.

'You ask too many questions for a patient. You might bleed when we take off the dressings.'

I meet him directly in the eyes and he looks away. I know he is not telling the truth but inside me a voice urges silence 'It's not the appointed time' – the words flood into my mind from nowhere. The question forming on my lips dies and I look at the young doctor again. He smiles awkwardly.

'Okay, Jimmy,' I reply instead. He relaxes visibly – and I feel a wave of fear flood over me.

'Get a good night's sleep now, won't you,' he advises, leaving my room.

When he has gone the silence is heavy and oppressive. I know something is going on and I feel bewildered and lonely. Closing my eyes I try

16

to pray, but the words will not form. 'Jesus,' I whisper. 'I am scared, so scared. Please help me.' I lie back against the pillow and close my eyes against the troubling world. The nurses bring me my tablets and I gulp them down eagerly. I want to be asleep and away from my anxiety. I pray quietly to myself and repeat over and over again the words that I have read in the Bible: 'Be not afraid, be not afraid.' Soon the fear is swallowed up in sleep.

I awake suddenly and, despite the heavy dose of sleeping tablets and painkillers, I am immediately alert. I am filled with a sense of expectancy. The room is becoming light and soon I am bathed in the brightest, purest light I have ever known. I know there is a physical presence in the right-hand corner of the room. The Presence is very tall and strong, reaching almost to the ceiling. For a few seconds I wait fearlessly as I know, somehow, that I am not in danger. I become aware of a deep peace filling me and I feel warm and joyful inside. The Presence moves towards me and instinctively I shuffle to one side to make more room. He sits on the edge of my bed and I am awe-struck by his physical size and strength. Suddenly I feel very, very safe. The peace within me becomes more and more overwhelming and streams of silent tears roll down my cheeks. Unexpectedly, sounds begin to form in my mouth. I do not know what language this is, so strange and unfamiliar, but I cannot seem to stop it. The words soothe me completely. They form clearly in my mind and I know they are being spoken to me directly by the Presence. Who or what is he? I do not know, but he is not of this world.

'Mary, I will lead you through the valley of the shadow of death,' the Presence says, 'but do not fear any evil, for I *will* bring you through.'

I know the words to be true and I sleep deeply and peacefully, sensing I am being watched over. When I wake I am aware that today, Friday 7 January, is to be a day like no other. I recall the previous night's experiences completely, calmly and naturally. I have glimpsed another spiritual realm, more powerful than any earthly state, and I wait for something to happen.

My room remains quiet for several hours, the usual hubbub of breakfast being denied me because of my visit to the operating theatre. A little later there is a tap on the door and Mr Peach enters. As soon as my eyes meet his I know something is wrong. He sits on my bed, exactly where the Presence sat, and takes my hand in his. I look at him trustingly.

'Well, Little Lady.' He speaks softly. 'You must be brave. That old lump – well, it was a nasty old thing.'

17

'What do you mean?'

'I'm afraid the lump was cancer.'

My world stops. I turn my head away, my mind searching frantically, desperately, for an alternative.

'Oh, God, no, not cancer.'

'There is an operation we could do. It wouldn't guarantee anything – but it would give you a chance.'

'What sort of operation?' I ask hesitantly, unable to imagine anything more extreme than what I have already undergone.

'We could remove your leg.' The words fall out cautiously.

'My leg? You would take my leg? My whole leg?'

Mr Peach nods. His eyes, holding mine, cry with me.

'Yes, my Little Lady,' he whispers. 'We need to amputate your leg.' His hand holds mine tightly and I draw strength from him.

In a moment's silence I contemplate all I had planned. My whole future: becoming a doctor, marrying, bearing children. In a few anguished seconds I see my world collapse.

'How can I still be a doctor? With one leg? Is it possible?'

Mr Peach looks at me thoughtfully as he balances hope and realism.

'It is possible … I have a friend, an orthopaedic surgeon. His leg was amputated because of cancer.'

'And if I don't have it? What then?'

'If we don't operate you will certainly die.'

Time stands still as I take it in.

'And …' I pause. 'Will I live if my leg is taken?'

'Possibly. There's a chance at least. You will need to have chemotherapy, though.'

I have heard about chemotherapy. My friend's sister nursed on a leukaemia ward and she told us about drugs that make patients bald and infertile.

'If I have chemotherapy, will my hair fall out?'

'Yes, every last hair.'

'And will I be infertile?'

'Yes, my dear,' he replies carefully. 'You will not be able to have children.'

I consider the options, minutes seeming like hours.

'Shall we operate then?' Mr Peach asks me.

'Yes, take my leg. I don't want to die. I'll be okay, you'll see.'

He assents gravely and looks at me. 'It's a brave decision, Mary, but I would choose the same.'

'And I will be a doctor, Mr Peach.'

He is visibly relieved the decision is made.

'I believe you,' he says, 'I truly believe you.'

'Shall we pray, Mr Peach?' He looks surprised.

'Yes, let's do that. Let's pray I will do a good job and you will get through all this.'

So the surgeon and the patient hold hands and pray the Lord's prayer together. 'Thy kingdom come, Thy will be done, on earth …'

Even as I say the words I wonder: 'Surely this is not Your will, for I cannot believe that?'

'Your mum and dad are outside, Mary,' Mr Peach tells me, and I panic.

Now I realize why my family didn't visit the previous day. They were at home, being told the awful news.

'But how will they ever cope with this?' I ask, knowing their dreams for me will also be shattered.

'They are strong, Little Lady, like you.' I agree, trustingly, willing to place everything into the hands of somebody strong and capable.

Mum and Dad enter the tiny airless room. I feel guilty; guilty that I have brought all this sadness upon them. Mum walks over to the window, tears blurring her unseeing vision. Dad sits on the bed and squeezes my hand too tight. They speak but I cannot hear them. I talk but I do not know what I say. They cry a lot and I realize I have never seen my dad cry before. They reassure me and tell me things will turn out but I feel older than them.

Falteringly I begin, 'I know about my leg. I have cancer. It is serious. I could die. They say they will take my leg and I can't have children and my hair will fall out.'

But then I add: 'You know that stuff about God and all that? Well, I still believe it.'

Strangely, as well, I do. I know I have already glimpsed beyond the grave.

'I will miss my leg,' I say simply. There is no other way to tell it.

A little later, I say goodbye to it. I reach forward and strain to touch my foot, the only part of my leg not covered in bandages. I tickle my big toe.

But God always answers prayers and God can do anything, say the priests. Does that mean maybe I won't have to lose my leg? I can still pray for a miracle. The cancer might disappear. Yes, that's it, I decide.

God will glorify Himself by transforming the cancer. All things are possible, the Bible says, and I believe those words. I have to, for the alternative is unthinkable.

I am given a tablet. I feel sleepy, so sleepy. I am wheeled down a corridor. I look up and see my dad striding alongside. It is cold and draughty and I see bright lights above me. A kind man talks to me and lifts up a syringe. As I drift into unconscious blackness, crying, I feel a finger reach over and tickle my toes. I believe with every fibre of my being that, when I wake up, my leg will still remain.

I awake into a world of silence. It is pitch black. I think I am dead. Then I remember the surgery. I strain to become aware of some bodily sensation. I try to focus my mind.

'Where are my hands?' I think, and I feel them. Slowly and heavily, I lift them. They are like lead weights. I reach down towards my leg but then another hand catches mine and restrains me. I do not fight, for I cannot. I let my arms flop down on the bed. My brain is beginning to work again.

'My leg, how does it feel?' I wonder. Then I become aware of a tickle on my left foot; it is my big toe. Yes, I can definitely feel it! My leg is still there. I concentrate with all my power. Every inch of my leg is there; toes, heel, knee and thigh. I feel the reassuring pressure of my heel on the mattress and the blankets touching the tip of my toe, the throbbing pain in my knee and the biting metal of the Thomas Splint.

'Thank you, God,' I pray. 'Thank you that the miracle worked and I still have my leg!' I drift back into the most wonderful of dreams, smiling.

When I open my eyes again the dawn is breaking and a pale light fills the room. Mum and Dad have been here day and night for me but, at this instant, I am alone. The figure who sat with me through the night is gone. I remember my leg has been cured. I can feel it, warm and still beside my good one. I try to move it … but it seems to be paralysed for some reason. Perhaps, I think, it is fastened to a splint. I reach down with my hand to explore. I put my hand on my thigh but I feel the cotton of the sheets. Blindly, I grope around but I cannot find my leg. I strain and lift my head, and see the truth.

I can hear a voice screaming and screaming. I wonder whose it is and then I realize it is mine. A nurse runs to me.

'My leg! Where is my leg?' I scream and do not stop until my mother steps back into the room and her kind voice breaks into my terror.

'Mary,' she sobs, 'your leg is gone.'

'But I can feel it, I know it's there!'

She says gently: 'That's not really your leg. It is your phantom leg. It is a trick of your mind.'

This mental torture is more agonizing than anything I will ever know again – anguish at the deception of my own body. I have no leg now, only a sensation of one. I want to feel nothing. I do not want a reminder of all I have lost. Even the tumour pain still mocks me; the evil Limpet which caused this grief still reminds me of its presence. Not so much pain, more the suggestion of pain. Worse than pain. Impossible to put into words.

'The miracle,' I whisper to my mum but she can't hear me. She smoothes my forehead with a cold damp cloth. She shakes her head, not understanding.

'It didn't work, Mum. The miracle didn't happen after all.'

3

This is the first day I have had any time to myself since the awful moment I woke up and discovered the miracle had failed. I feel as if I am living in another world, a world that I don't want to be in. People come and go in my room and I talk to them but I cannot remember what I have said. I smile and nod, I even pray with them, but it cannot be me. I feel numb, detached and unreal. I am living in a horrible dream and soon I will wake up again. They tell me I am brave and my faith is an inspiration but I do not even know what I am saying. I don't want to be brave; I want to be whole. I don't want to be an inspiration; I would rather be beautiful.

If I lie here with my eyes closed, I can feel my left leg – every inch of it. I am keeping my eyes closed so I don't have to be in this world where terrible things happen. I can pretend I am somewhere, anywhere, just as long as I have my leg back. Two days have gone by now and I have not looked under the sheets yet. The nurses come and fuss, changing dressings and pulling at the tubes draining my bladder and my wounds. Dr Jimmy hangs up bags of blood to run through my drip and I watch the bright red fluid feeding me back to life, a life that I no longer recognize.

'You're looking better,' they say to me. I want to scream at them.

'No, I am never going to look better,' I want to say.

Today is Monday 10 January 1983. They took my leg on Friday. I cannot remember Saturday. I kept drifting in and out of sleep. Sometimes I woke up and thought my leg was there and then, other times, I knew it wasn't. My mum was always there for me, holding me like a baby and stroking my hair. I remember she pulled my hands away time and time again when I tried to explore my damaged body. Except it is not my body any more; I do not recognize it. Yesterday I woke up a little bit more but, when I did, I wanted to be asleep again because it was hurting so much. Pains as sharp as hot pins started to shoot down my missing leg from hip to toe and what is left of it started to jump with a life of its own.

I was so scared and frightened and I began to cry. Dr Jimmy came and explained it is caused by the nerves beginning to learn that my leg is no longer there. He weighted my stump down with some little bags of sand. He asked me if I wanted to look at it but I couldn't. I don't want to see it, ever. I am just going to lie here and pretend my leg is still there.

Yesterday I had loads of visitors. My best friend, Adele, surprised me by turning up. She is stunning-looking: blonde, tall and leggy. I told her I felt ugly and she is going to help me feel better about that. She promised to bring me in some pretty nightdresses and then she brushed my hair for me. She actually said it looked as if the poison was out of my body. She said I looked healthier already. I guess in a way she is right; I suppose the cancer was poisoning me. But I have been wondering if maybe it would have been better to be poisoned.

I asked Dr Jimmy how long the jumping and the pains would go on for. He said it could take a long time and the phantom feelings might always stay with me. He said I will get used to it and adapt, but I can't see how. It is really annoying me that I cannot cross my feet. I keep moving as if to, and then I realize the phantom leg can't move. It is paralysed. Normally, I can feel my two knees gently touching each other and lying there side by side like two good friends. Now there is only one knee in the bed. I want to cry, I want to shout and scream, but I can't; I feel frozen. It is as if time inside has stopped and everything else around me is carrying on.

When I get the pains I ask the nurses for an injection. It hurts when they do it but then it makes me feel lovely, all floaty and dreamy. Nothing seems to matter to me then, not even my missing leg. I feel extraordinarily happy after it so I ask the nurses for the injection as often as I can. It is like lying on a cloud and it makes me laugh a lot. They also give me tablets which just make me relax and sleep, so I can lie here and dream away and not have to think about the real world. I think I will stay here for as long as I can.

Because it was Sunday yesterday, loads of priests came to see me. It looked a bit like Vatican City. One of the older ones brought me Communion and said a prayer but it sounded hollow. He prayed for me to be strengthened instead of healed. I don't want to be strengthened; I want my leg back. I do not understand why the miracle didn't work despite the fact that everybody prayed so hard for healing. I was convinced God was going to save my leg. I thought God always heard our prayers. I have so many questions and no answers. When I ask the priests they say there is a purpose behind it all. They say God uses suffering. I don't want to be used any more. If I pray hard enough I know I will have my leg back. That would be the second miracle. Hopefully it will happen soon. I know I am going to walk out of here on two healthy legs. Then the cancer will disappear, which will be the third miracle. Then everybody will believe in God – they would have to, if a leg grew back. That is probably why God has done this to me! Yes, that is His purpose. He is going to use me, just as I asked that day in the church in the Lake District.

Mum and Dad have been with me around the clock since the amputation. I cannot bear to see them crying and so sad. I have been trying to tell them God is going to heal me but somehow it seems to make them feel worse. I need to be strong for them so they don't get hurt any more. I want to be brave so they will be happy again. I feel guilty because I have made them so upset. They ask me how I am and I say I am all right because I hate to see them this worried. And I will be all right, once I get my leg back.

I am awoken from my daydreams by a knock on the door. It is early in the morning, so it can't be more visitors. Mr Peach enters my room.

'Hello, my brave Little Lady,' he greets me, and immediately I feel better. 'How is my star patient?'

I want to please him and bask in his admiration, for he is my hero.

'I'm fine,' I say, and smile.

'How is your pain today?'

'It's not very nice. I can feel my leg as if it's still there and I keep feeling as if somebody is pricking it with sharp pins. Dr Jimmy told me the pains might be around for a long time.' I wait for him to answer, holding my breath. Maybe Jimmy got it wrong.

'Yes, it's true,' he agrees. 'Phantom legs sometimes stay for life, although the unpleasant sensations will hopefully get less.'

'But how can I live with it? It's so strange!'

'I know it sounds unbelievable now,' he explains, slowly, 'but your mind will adapt. Lots of amputees say they just learn to ignore their phantoms.'

I find it hard to believe that I will ever be able to ignore the ghost of my leg and then I remember with a rush of relief that I won't have to, once the second miracle works.

'God is going to heal me, Mr Peach,' I say seriously. He looks at me cautiously.

'Mary, it will take time to adjust to losing your leg. It's a bit like losing somebody you love. You will need time to grieve.'

I laugh nonchalantly and say, 'Okay, Mr Peach.' Inside I know he will be amazed at what will happen. I can't wait to see his face when my leg has grown back. I decide not to tell him because I don't think he believes in God. It will be great, though, when he is converted by the miracle. How pleased the God Squad will be, too.

He goes on to explain what will happen next.

'The operation is over, Mary, but there is a lot of work to be done now. We need to get you up and about, so we have to start some physiotherapy to help you learn to balance and strengthen your muscles. First of all, we need to get you sitting upright again.'

'Well, that's not difficult is it?' I ask him curiously.

I have been lying flat on my back for two weeks now and I can't wait to sit up again. This view of the ceiling is getting dull!

'Let's try, then, shall we?' He laughs and his strong arms lift me off the pillow for a few seconds so I am sitting upright. The room begins to lurch crazily and my head is in a spin.

'Help!' I cry. 'Put me down!'

'Your body has to learn to walk and balance all over again.'

'It's like being on a ship! How long will it be like this?'

'We will sit you up a little bit each day, beginning tomorrow, and then maybe by the end of the week we can get you out into a chair.'

I sink back on my soft pillows, exhausted. He turns to the nurse and issues further instructions.

'Drip and catheter out tomorrow, Sister.' He waves to me and is gone.

I replay the conversation. 'I must not doubt,' I think to myself. 'God will give me back my leg so I won't need stupid physiotherapy.' I close my eyes and return to my little fantasy world.

Some time later I open my eyes and see Hellie sitting beside me. Because of the pain and the anaesthetic, I have not been able to talk to her since the operation. She is dressed in her school uniform and I remember it is the first day of a new term. Her eyes are bright with unshed tears.

25

'Hello, Big Sis,' and she gives me a hug. It feels so good to be held close to a warm, healthy body. 'I've missed you.'

'I missed you, too.'

'I love you, Mary.'

'I love you, too.' We hug again and laugh. We hug so much, she knocks the cupboard by the side of the bed. There is a huge crash and water, flowers and glass end up all over the floor. We look at each other, Hellie and I, our eyes wide with alarm. Time is frozen, for so much is broken. I cannot decide if I should laugh or cry and I check out my sister's reaction.

'Whoops!' she says slowly. We laugh until we cry, the tears rolling down our cheeks, and a nurse comes in to tell Hellie off.

'I am so glad to see you at last,' Hellie says. 'You don't know what it's been like!'

'Tell me, I want to know.'

She looks at me and rolls her eyes. 'Everyone has been upset and crying.'

'When did you find out about my leg?' I ask her.

'Thursday night. Mr Peach came to see Mum and Dad and they spent ages talking. I heard Mum crying. Then, when he left, Mum and Dad told Martin and me. Adrian doesn't know yet – he's away on holiday, remember? He comes back tomorrow.'

'What about Franny?' I ask, recalling that she is away at college.

'Pastor Tony told Franny. She's coming to see you this weekend. Tony has been really fantastic, ringing Mum and Dad every day. Of course, everybody is praying at church and the priests are helping Mum and Dad. They are clinging on to their faith.'

'Hellie, does Martyn know yet?' I have been thinking about him a lot and wondering who told him. He will feel guilty, I know.

She looks at me hesitantly. 'No-one told him. He found out in assembly this morning. Mr McCarthy announced about your illness. Martyn walked out of the hall.'

'Oh no!' I feel a pang of pain and compassion for him and, looking away, I fight back more tears.

'Anyway, I'm here to cheer you up,' she says briskly, handing me a tiny package.

'What's this for?'

'It's from the folk group, the God Squad, everyone – go on, open it.'

I open the neatly wrapped package to find a gold bracelet and pretty tins of make-up. I look for a few seconds, bewildered, not knowing what to do next.

'Right, my girl, time to do your make-up! You are going to look great when I've finished with you!' She works silently on my face and hair for a few minutes, then sits back and looks at me.

'You look gorgeous, you know,' she says to me. 'I'm being serious. You kind of have this inner peace. It shines through your eyes.'

'But I feel so ugly, Hellie,' I confess softly. 'My body feels … damaged, mutilated.'

Her eyes hold mine and she is angry. 'No, Mary! You mustn't say that, ever! You are *not* ugly, do you hear me? You have to believe me! It doesn't matter that you don't have your leg. You are still beautiful. You are just different!'

'But I hate being different. I don't want to be different.'

'Okay then, you are special.'

'I don't want to be special. I want to be ordinary.'

She holds up the mirror for me, exasperated. I have not looked in a mirror for several days. I close my eyes.

'Open your eyes, Mary. Look! I haven't done your make-up for nothing.'

I do as I am told. I am stunned. My face is the same – oval, freckled, just a little thinner. My eyes are the same clear blue. Nothing has changed. Except my leg and, with it, my life.

'Okay, Miss Beautiful,' she jokes. 'I hope those Ward Six boys come to visit you, especially the good-looking one! Barry, is it?' I had mentioned my new friends while Hellie worked.

I blush and she laughs as she leaves the room, waving goodbye and promising to visit me every day.

The room is unbearably quiet afterwards. Is it possible that I can still be considered beautiful after what has been done to me? I cannot see how anyone will ever be able to look at me and love me again. I do not feel whole any more. I have always been strong and healthy. I am the one who wins the athletics races and makes the sports teams. I love to dance and turn cartwheels. Now all I can do is lie in a bed. I think about so many problems in the future – how can I possibly learn to walk if I cannot even sit up unaided?

I try to sleep but I am burdened with a heavy heart. Thoughts of easier days go round and round. I imagine myself running down mountains and leaping through rivers. I feel trapped inside a useless body. The phantom pains remind me again and again of a lifetime to come – however brief it might be – of pain and loss. My fear escalates and I begin to panic. I ring the nurses' bell and a worried staff nurse appears. 'What's wrong, Mary?' she asks.

'I can't sleep. It hurts. Everything hurts.' I just want out of this frightening world. I want everyone to leave me alone.

'Okay, love. We'll sort it for you.' She sticks a needle in my good thigh and helps me take a tablet. Soon I descend into a tunnel of blackness and glorious silence …

The last few days have been awful. I do not quite understand how I have got where I am. It is now almost a week since my amputation. The days have settled into a routine. It is still horrible, but at least I know what to expect. There are not so many nasty surprises.

Each day Mr Peach asks the nurses to sit me up a little more. Now I am upright and can move around the bed on my own. One by one the various tubes have been taken out of my body: first the drip, then the catheter, then the tubes draining my wounds. It hurt a lot when Mr Peach took those out. In fact I screamed and swore. Now they are all gone and I am left with a bandaged stump. The pains are still there, shooting like lightning, but my phantom has changed. Instead of a strong and healthy ghost leg, it is now swollen and mis-shapen. It feels as if I have a gigantic foot and a short leg. But at least I know it isn't real. I am learning to push it out of my mind. Every day the physiotherapist comes to see me. Over the week she has made me sit up and close my eyes and try and stay upright. At first I was swaying all over the place but now I am quite steady. She helps me do special exercises. She pummels and pushes me and I feel really tired. She tells me I need to strengthen my muscles so I can learn to walk again. She bandages my stump and tells me I will learn to do this so I can use an artificial limb. But I turn my head away and refuse to look at my mutilated body. What none of them realize is that I will not need to do all this. I am just going along with it until my leg grows back.

Every day I check under the bedclothes to see if it is there yet. It seems to be taking some time. I want Mr Peach to be the first person to know about the miracle so I always check first thing when I wake up. So far it has not happened but I am not giving up faith. I must continue to trust and I know God will use all things for good. I just wish He would hurry up and get me out of this hospital so I can spread the word.

My mum and dad visit every day. Mum is very strong and brings me lovely surprises. She has stopped crying and instead tells me all the news and chats. She and Hellie have been shopping to buy me new clothes. Things I can wear without my leg. She brought some of them in to show me and, of course, they are so fashionable because Hellie chose them. I told her not to throw my tight jeans away, though. Mum seemed a little puzzled when I said that. But then miracles don't happen in our church. This will be the first. She is going to be amazed when it happens to me! Dad usually comes to see me on his way home from work. He is silent and worried. I don't think he believes I am going to be healed. Hellie comes to see me at lunchtime and fills me in on the school gossip. She seems to have grown older in the last few days. My little brother Adrian is so upset he will not speak to anybody.

When my friends visit me from school, I tell them it's okay. I tell them God is using me for His glory. I smile this big smile. I call it my plaster saint smile. But all they do is cry or sit there and ask dumb questions. It feels as if they are children and I am no longer part of their world. And yet I would far rather be part of their world. I don't want to be here. I wish I could run away. But, of course, I can't run anywhere now. I read my Bible and my prayer book and I talk about miracles and things like that. I pretend I am amazingly happy because of being close to God. Everybody tells me I am so brave. My faith is very strong, they say, and I'm an inspiration. How can I tell them that sometimes I don't even believe in God now, let alone heaven, and I am just so scared of it hurting? It already hurts. My leg and my hip and all the injections. I guess dying from cancer must take ages and it must really, really hurt. Where is God? Where is He? Heaven? What is it like? I don't want to be stuck on a cloud with a pair of wings and loads of old people. It sounds pretty boring. I read this bit about heaven in the Bible – the book of Revelation. It was like reading Shakespeare on a bad day. It was going on about golden lampstands and walls made of jasper, white horses and red dragons and seas made of glass. And do you know what I thought? I thought it sounded horrible. Scary and weird. I don't want to go somewhere like that. I'd rather stay here with my sisters and my school lessons and my pretty clothes.

But today I feel quite excited because I get to sit up in the armchair and, if I do that, then I can use a wheelchair. It has taken a whole week even to achieve this tiny step. I feel nervous about getting out of bed. I have been here now for three long weeks since I was admitted on

Boxing Day. It also means I will have to look at my body – and my stump. I still haven't done that. I am filled with a sense of expectancy as my favourite nurse arrives with the physiotherapist.

'Ready for the big moment?' she jokes.

I nod and sit up. 'You bet!' I say enthusiastically. 'I can't wait to get out of here.'

'No guesses for where you'll be going first!' she teases. Barry from Ward Six has been to visit me a couple of times.

The first time I saw the Ward Six boys after my operation was really difficult. The door crashed open and Peter yelled, 'Surprise again!' and in they all came in their wheelchair convoy. Of course, the thing they all noticed was that my splint had gone.

'What happened, then?' asked Peter, who is a bit vague after his head injury.

I realized with horror that they didn't know about my amputation. I felt sick with fear at the thought of telling them. I stammered and tripped over my words. It was the first time I had needed to tell anyone myself. 'Well, I had to … I had to …' and stopped.

I looked in shock towards Barry, beseeching him to understand.

'Are you okay, Mary?' he asked, and I shook my head and felt the hot tears well up again. 'Right you two – out!' he ordered.

'Tell me what they did, Mary,' he said gently.

'I can't,' I whispered. 'It's too awful.'

'They took your leg, didn't they? You have cancer, yes?'

I nodded slowly and he wheeled over and held my hand.

'Oh kid, I'm so sorry,' he said, and I wished everyone could be as understanding as him.

So since then he has been to visit me and I love his easy smile and his stories of falling off bikes. I guess he is just being kind.

'Hey, Mary, come on,' urges the nurse. 'Stop daydreaming and start practising and then you can go and visit lover-boy!' We laugh. I was miles away.

'Swing your leg round in the bed so you are sitting on the edge.' She lowers the bed for me.

'Okay, now put your foot on the floor nice and firmly.' She pauses and lets me get used to the feeling of planting my one and only foot on the floor for the first time. It feels weird. I keep wanting to put the other one next to it. I stretch out my leg and look at my toes and count them out loud.

'One, two, three, four, five!' I look at the nurse. 'There should be ten, you know. One day there will be.'

I spend a moment looking critically at the little bulge under the hem of my night dress. 'And there will be two feet and two knees.'

'No, Mary, that won't happen. Your leg has gone – you know that. You will always have five toes, one foot, one knee.'

'No, they will grow back. Just wait and see.'

'Mary,' she says firmly. 'Look at me.'

I glance at her from beneath my fringe, sulkily.

'No, properly.'

I sigh and look at her.

'Mary, your leg is not coming back. Not one day. Not ever.'

As I stare into her eyes my veil of deception drops and suddenly, with the force of a ten-ton truck, I am hit with the dreadful realization. I cry out in pain and I throw the pillow across the room.

'No! no! It's not going to happen! My leg is gone!' I collapse in a pile on the bed and my body is racked by huge heaving sobs as my mind takes in, for the first time, the full scale of the damage.

'Why, why?' I cry out time and time again and we are all weeping. The nurse holds me close and rocks me like a baby. Soon her uniform is soaked with my tears.

'Shh, there, there.' She soothes me and strokes my hair. 'You've been so strong. We were waiting for this. Have a good cry. Cry it all out.' So I cry for what seems like hours. I cry out all the pain and fear, the frustration and the disappointment. I shout at the unfairness of it all and the destruction of my hopes and the devastation of my plans. Most of all I rage at the mutilation of my body, my beautiful strong body. I hate the Limpet for doing this. I hate it for ever.

After I am all cried away, the nurses leave and I lie on my bed in agony. I feel abandoned. 'Please God, help me,' I pray softly, not expecting an answer. I now know what it is to feel utter despair. I wait silently and mutter to myself, 'Help me, help me.'

In the silence after the storm I feel a peace descend. It starts in my chest and spreads out, a warmth filling me. It is as if I am being held in a giant hand. I curl up further and whimper but I am not scared. I am back to being a baby. I feel caressed and soothed and I become aware of God being close to me. I remember the words of the Presence, 'I will lead you through the valley of the shadow of death,' and I try to think what came next. 'But I will bring you through.'

31

I surrender to an overwhelming desire to sleep. When I awake the anger is gone and the fear is replaced with a calm knowledge that I will never be alone again. Somewhere in the darkness and despair I can still find a distant glimpse of my God.

Mr Peach arrives to see me later in the afternoon.

'Hello, Little Lady,' he greets me. 'I hear you've had a bad time.'

'Yes, but I feel better now.'

'I can understand that. It's a slow process coming to terms with this at such a young age. You've had to grow up very quickly.' He smiles at me and adds: 'You are doing very well, you know. So well that you can have a wheelchair to get around in. I want you to practise this weekend. Next week we need to begin your tests, and it would speed things up a lot if we can get you up and about.'

'Tests?'

'We need to check that the cancer from your bone has not got into your system. So we will do some tests to check out the rest of your body. Apart from the pain in your leg, you haven't had any other symptoms, so that is a very good sign.'

'So if the tests are clear, what does that mean?'

'We will send you to another hospital for chemotherapy.'

'And where will that be?'

'The Christie Hospital in Manchester.'

I feel anxious again. I didn't realize I would be away from home but I like the sound of the hospital. I imagine it as being kind and benevolent.

'How long will it all take?'

Mr Peach looks at me cautiously and I know I do not want to hear his answer.

'A long time, I'm afraid.' I steel myself again. 'Two years.'

'Two years? In hospital? I can't go through that!'

'You will be able to have times at home.'

I consider the options. I should be starting to live my life, taking my A levels, going to university. I can't just sit in a hospital.

'What if I don't have the chemotherapy?'

'If you don't have the chemotherapy then I'm afraid that you will not get better.'

'You mean I will die?' I meet his gaze again.

'Yes, that's what I mean.' I am glad he is honest.

'And if the tests aren't clear?'

He drops his eyes and looks at his hands. 'Let's cross that bridge when we come to it, shall we?'

He thinks I have heard enough, but I know anyway. I will die if the tests aren't clear. So I sigh and ask, 'What tests do I need?' He tells me I will have to undergo a bone scan, a full body CT scan and some X-rays, and they will start on Monday.

'So get a good weekend's rest, in between practising your driving!'

I am left wondering how much more I have to take. I had managed to push the thought of the cancer away while I was recovering from my surgery and now I have to face it again. I worry all day and hardly listen when my mum comes to visit and outlines the arrangements for my stay in Manchester. I look at her and notice she has lost weight and there are dark shadows under her eyes.

'Your teachers have promised to come in and see you so you won't fall behind with your work too badly.' I feel depressed, thinking of so much wasted time. I want to be home with my brother and sister and my books. I want my pretty bedroom and my cuddly toys.

When Mum goes I pray again. I am confused. What am I doing wrong? Why are all these awful things happening to me? I am scared of dying. I am only seventeen. 'How long until I die?' I think to myself. I haven't even begun to live my life. I am only a child. I haven't done anything, seen anything, lived anything yet. Time, time that uncertain commodity. It is time I crave. I am so young, so young. I didn't know seventeen-year-olds could die of cancer. Maybe it is my fault. Perhaps I have done something terribly wrong to deserve this punishment. I know God loves me. But if He loves me then why am I so ill? Maybe I got ill because of what I did with Martyn – maybe I went too far. Maybe that's why God has taken my beauty away. My life seems so fragile and uncertain now. It is as though the dark chasm of death is always before me.

I am scared; very scared.

4

My tests have started. They are looking for secondaries. And I must learn to fight this death to the death. I now understand a little more about what is happening inside my body. The cancer is spreading. The cells are in my blood, waiting to find a place to rest. They may even have settled down to suck out my life already. Perhaps at this very second they are getting tired of whizzing round my veins and arteries and are deciding to put down roots. If I have any other tumours then I will die. If I pray hard enough then maybe the cancer will not spread and the secondaries will die and I will live. Maybe I will escape the chemotherapy, too. This is the third miracle. The first two miracles failed, keeping my leg and then my leg growing back. I am sure this one will work; it has to. I cannot imagine God wants me to die. What would be the sense in that? I have so much to do with my life. I have the message to spread and people to convert. I cannot do that if I am dead. I guess this miracle is a bit easier than the other two. Getting rid of the Limpet and growing a leg back – well, they were pretty difficult miracles. Killing the other tumours should be a lot easier.

Over the weekend I practised getting around in my wheelchair and learnt how to get in and out of it myself. This is called a wheelchair transfer and it is exhausting. I need to lift my entire weight with my arms, which leaves my muscles quivering. But I feel proud to have regained this little bit of independence. I can do things like go and chat to the nurses and wheel up and down the corridor. It will be great when I am allowed to go and visit Ward Six on my own! Barry is back on his splint because he has re-fractured his leg. Just Peter and Steve come to see me now, and they make me laugh, but it is not the same without Barry. I miss him a lot.

Franny came to see me on Sunday with Pastor Tony. I haven't seen her since the operation. We both cried a lot at first. Then, as she's a physiotherapist, I asked her a lot of questions about getting an artificial leg. I was wondering how real they look, and she told me they look very much like proper legs and I will be able to wear normal clothes and shoes. I felt a lot better, knowing they look realistic. I had imagined going round with a wooden peg and looking really peculiar.

We all prayed together and Pastor Tony gave me some little cards with scripture verses on them so I don't have to spend hours looking for them in my Bible. They helped me. They said not to be afraid because Jesus is looking after me and, for a moment, I could almost remember how I felt before the Limpet struck. Back then it was easy to believe Jesus was looking out for me. Now I am not quite so sure. I mean, Jesus never had a problem doing miracles in His day but now it seems to be taking for ever. In the small hours of the morning, when I am alone, sometimes I think the miracle will not happen at all.

On Monday I went for my chest X-rays. Mr Peach seemed quite worried about my lungs. I asked Dr Jimmy why this was and he explained that if the cancer spreads it would go there first. It was very important that this first test was clear. A nurse took me down in my wheelchair and I felt absolutely free! It was also the first time, with my new and ungainly body, that I was meeting people I didn't know. The nurse pushed me along the corridor and I passed a lady with a small child. The pretty girl looked at me with wide puzzled eyes and I overheard the mother telling her not to stare. With a shock I realized she was talking about me. I cringed, not so much at the curiosity of a four-year-old, but rather at the mother's reprimanding whisper. It drew more attention to me, making me feel even more embarrassed and awkward.

It didn't take long for the X-rays to be taken, so my trip to freedom was short-lived. On the return journey I asked the nurse for a blanket to cover my solitary leg. For the first time I had discovered how painful it is to be different.

Mr Peach came to see me a bit later and jovially entered my room.

'It's great news, Little Lady!' he greeted me. 'The X-rays are clear. Your lungs are fine. That is a very good sign.'

I was so relieved. It was the first good news I had received.

'So what does it mean, then?'

'Well, it's a good indication that your lungs are free of any spread from the bone tumour so we can go ahead and do the other tests which are more sensitive.'

He appeared overjoyed and I realized he hadn't been expecting the tests to be clear.

'Tomorrow we will do a CT scan of your whole body, which will give us more information,' he added.

'I told you that God would heal me, didn't I?' I said, and Mr Peach smiled at me.

'Yes, you did say that, and it looks as if God is listening to your prayers!'

The test result gave me confidence. I spent some time putting on my make-up, styling my hair and donning my favourite nightdress. A round of applause greeted me as I pushed myself triumphantly down the length of Ward Six.

'Hey, look who's here!' shouted Peter. The boys gathered round me in their wheelchairs and Barry waved from his bed.

'You made it then, kid!' he quipped and we all wheeled over to his bedside. I told my friends about the test results and they were delighted.

'This calls for a celebration,' said Peter and signalled to Barry for his jug of water. I noticed there were three glasses on his bedside table.

'Get a glass for Mary,' urged Barry. I wondered what they were up to. Barry poured four small glasses and handed them to us. The boys winked at me and said in unison, 'Cheers!' They all seemed very jolly. I took a sip and, as I swallowed, the back of my throat burned.

'Vodka!' whispered Peter and we all laughed together. I felt accepted and safe, for we were all different here. After a few minutes Steve and Peter disappeared, leaving me with Barry. We talked for a while until a nurse came to tell me that I needed to let him rest. As I left, Barry blew me a kiss and I blushed.

'You look lovely when you blush,' he said to me and I left the ward with my heart singing.

I was on a cloud of dreams for the rest of the day and the nurses teased me. I felt normal again and it was wonderful. I have tapes of Beatles love ballads and I listened to them all day. By the evening, I was in love. I pushed myself dreamily down to the bathroom to get ready for bed, then lay there cuddling my teddy bear. I thought about Barry and, for a moment, I felt like a beautiful teenager again. Then I remembered what lay ahead of me the following day and I felt a pit of fear swallowing my fantasy. I wondered if I would ever know again the safety and innocence of being a carefree child.

Yesterday was Tuesday and I had my CT scan. I felt very nervous about it. I knew it was crucial for it to be clear. Everyone was tense and on edge. The scanner is shaped like a huge circle with a hole in the middle and the bed slides through it slowly. A kind lady greeted me and pointed to a picture of a grinning cat on the door.

'This is our CAT scanner,' she laughed. 'We also call it the magic Polo mint.'

'Will you stay in the room with me?' I asked, feeling overwhelmed.

'I'm sorry, Mary, I have to stay in that little room because of the radiation. But we can see you from behind the glass and I can talk to you through a microphone.' She helped me up on to a narrow bed. She seemed so kind.

'Did you know that God is going to heal me?' She looked at me and smiled. She pointed to a little brooch on her collar in the shape of a dove.

'I'm a Christian too,' she said. 'Let's ask God to strengthen you and look after you, shall we?' I felt disappointed. I wanted a miracle.

'Can I keep my little cross with me?' I asked her.

'I'm such a spoilsport, aren't I?' she joked, but explained the metal would spoil the pictures.

'I'll be praying all the time you are in there,' she promised and squeezed my hand tightly before leaving. She waved to me from behind the glass screen but I couldn't wave back because my hands were strapped against my sides. I was all alone and scared. I wanted a hug from somebody. I wanted my mum and dad and tears sprang to my eyes. I was unable to wipe them and they trickled down the sides of my cheeks. The machine started to make a loud humming noise and then some clicks. It moved slowly over my head, so close that I could feel the metal touching my hair. I closed my eyes and tried to remember a verse of scripture.

'Be not afraid,' I thought to myself and repeated it like a mantra. 'Be not afraid.' I thought of the kind lady praying for me and I felt calmer.

It seemed like hours before the scanner reached my toes. Then the lady came in to help me sit up. She was smiling a lot. I got my little cross back.

'Was it okay?' I asked her.

'Well, officially I'm not allowed to tell you,' she said slowly but, seeing my anxious face, she added, 'Put it like this: I think your prayers are working.'

Mr Peach came bounding into my room as soon as I was back on the ward.

'The scan is clear! That's the best news that we can give you!' I was overjoyed. Mr Peach was happy, Dr Jimmy was happy, the nurses were happy. My mum and dad were ecstatic when they came to visit me later.

'You see!' I told them all, 'I told you God would heal me!'

There was an air of celebration all day. I told everybody about the miracle and they all commended my faith. I couldn't wait to tell the God Squad that I had been spreading the word. Perhaps now everybody would begin to believe and then my suffering would have been for a reason.

Now today, Wednesday, I have the last of my tests. It is the most sensitive of all. This time I am having a bone scan which involves an injection of a radioactive chemical, then afterwards they take some special pictures. If there are any tumours, even microscopic ones, they will glow brightly on the pictures. If they are clear then Mr Peach will contact Christie's and arrange for me to be transferred there for treatment.

If they are not clear … then I go home to die.

I hope I go to Christie's, but not too soon. I am beginning to enjoy so much being with Barry. Christie's is miles away. I will be away from Mum and Dad and so lonely. I feel safe here because everybody knows my dad and people pop in all the time. Two years seem to stretch into the future without any end in sight. It feels like the rest of my life.

When I get down to the X-ray department I am surprised to see Mr Peach holding a massive syringe enclosed in a big metal box and his hands encased in thick gloves.

'Is that for me?' I ask fearfully.

'Yes,' Mr Peach says, taking my hand and squeezing it. 'The metal box and the gloves are because of it being radio-active.' He finds a vein in my arm and injects the chemical into my body. Then he tells me to rest while they take the pictures. I feel very unwell, my head starts to spin and everything goes black. I wake up in my room. Dr Jimmy comes to see me.

'You fainted during the test, Mary,' he tells me. 'We will have to do another one tomorrow.'

He leaves the room and I hear him talking with the ward sister outside the door. I listen to snatches of words I don't understand – 'cerebral … metastases … convulsions … prognosis …' I feel terrified again.

What has happened to the miracle? Is something going wrong again? Why is everybody so concerned? Mr Peach comes to see me and I decide to ask him what 'metastases' means.

'It's another name for a secondary,' he tells me honestly. 'Where did you hear it?'

'I think I read it somewhere, on a test form maybe,' I lie, not wanting to get Jimmy into trouble. My heart lurches with despair when I realize Dr Jimmy was talking about secondaries in my brain. I didn't even know it could happen.

'So could I get secondaries anywhere, then?' I ask. Mr Peach looks at me thoughtfully, wondering how much he should tell me.

'Nearly always they are in the lungs,' he explains. 'But sometimes they can occur in other places.'

'And if they did?' I push him more, for I must find out what Jimmy was saying.

'Well … it would be very bad news indeed,' he says gravely.

I try to push away thoughts of the Limpet attacking my brain but I can't. Time and time again I return to the words. I think back over my life and worry about all the sins I have committed. I feel a sickening spasm of guilt and shame. My seventeen-year-old conscience decides I deserve to die. Please, God, don't let me die and please forgive me. I will do anything, but don't let me die.

I don't sleep at all, even with my tablets, and I am glad when the pale light of dawn fills the room. I am exhausted; there are dark shadows under my eyes and I am in pain. I hear a voice in my head.

'You would be better off, you know …'

I fight the voice of despair.

'What sort of future do you have? What about a window – you could break it and jump.' I am stunned at the clarity and the suddenness of the thought. I don't know where it came from.

'Just wheel along and break the glass while nobody is around and then …'

I think to myself that I couldn't break the glass and then, just as quickly, the voice interrupts my thoughts.

'What about the arm on your wheelchair – that would do the job.'

Ward Eight is at least three storeys up. It would be quick and easy. It would hurt but only, I guess, for a few seconds. I get out of bed and into the wheelchair. This is the only way to escape. I no longer know what is reality. I am so confused.

I wheel to the door as if in a dream. Nobody is about. I can hear the nurses laughing and joking in their office. I recognize Dr Jimmy's cheerful voice telling them about his busy night.

'God, if You are there and You love me, do something,' I pray angrily and despairingly, but also half-expecting nothing from Him. I turn right along the corridor and start to wheel myself slowly in the direction of a window.

The voice in my head reassures me. 'It will be okay. It will only hurt for a bit.'

I wonder where it has come from and think I must be going mad.

The voice is persuasive and smooth. 'Just one little jump and that will be it.'

As I approach the window, I see a figure in a wheelchair, silhouetted against the dawn light. I think it must be a ghost. 'It must be a sign,' I think to myself. Then the figure turns, lifts his hand and waves.

'Hi, Mary! What are you doing up so early?'

With a jolt I am catapulted out of my dreamlike state.

'Oh, hi Steve. I couldn't sleep. I decided to take a walk!' We laugh together.

'Me too,' he points towards the window. 'I often come here in the morning and watch the day beginning.' He looks at me and smiles, his head on one side. 'You know, Barry really likes you. He talks about you all the time. We all love you coming to see us in the ward.'

'What, me?' I ask incredulously.

'Yes, you! You give us all courage. We think you are amazingly brave and, although none of us believe in God … well, you've made us think.'

'Well, thanks.' I don't know what else to say but inside I feel proud and somehow worthy again. I tell Steve about the tests and he listens to my fears.

'You'll be okay, Mary,' he says. 'We all know you're going to get through this – remember that. We're counting on you!' We wheel back down the corridor together and, as we part company, I realize God answered my desperate prayer.

Entering the ward, I bump into Dr Jimmy.

'Hello, Mary,' he says brightly. 'Where have you been? You look as if you've seen a ghost!'

'I have!' I reply and, heaving myself on to my bed, I curl up. I am filled with a warm peace which makes me recall the Presence and I sleep deeply.

'Fantastic news!' rejoices Mr Peach later. 'The bone scan is clear.' It has been such a long day but now I have my answer. All the tests are clear. Mum and Dad are with me and I see them turn to each other and silently communicate. Everybody seems to breathe a huge collective sigh of relief.

'So what is the plan now?' I ask Mr Peach, eager to make more progress.

'We need to get you over to Christie's as soon as possible. I'll ring them straight away.'

Now I am left alone with Mum and Dad and we all give each other a big hug. After all the bad news, this is a little glimmer of light. I begin to think, 'Maybe, just maybe …'

Mr Peach returns quickly, smiling broadly.

'I have some very good news, Mary. I have just spoken with Dr Pearson — she is the consultant who will be looking after you. She tells me they are trying out a new regime of treatment. It is very intensive but it would only go on for three months and not two years as we expected. She thinks you would be a perfect patient for it.'

'Is it as good as the other type?' my dad asks.

'Yes. In fact, the results look even better. The only problem is that while Mary has the treatment she may be very ill.'

'I'll go for it,' I say. I have worked out I can still take my A levels, and the thought of shortening my hospital stay is so attractive.

'Will it still have the same side-effects?' I ask as an afterthought.

'Yes, it will,' replies Mr Peach.

'So, if I make it and if anyone wants to marry me, I will still be infertile?' My mum looks away and when she turns her head back I see she is crying.

'I'm afraid so. And it will still affect your lovely hair-do.'

'But I have a chance, at least?'

'Yes, it gives you a chance.'

'So when do I go?'

Mr Peach looks at me again. Strangely, I am not afraid today. Somehow, after my experience of despair this morning, I know that there is someone looking out for me.

'They want you there on Monday.'

'Oh, so soon!' I think of Barry and how much he means to me.

'It means you could be finished by May.' Mr Peach looks straight at me. He knows I am thinking about my A levels.

41

'Right then, I will go on Monday.'

He nods and adds, 'I thought that's what you would say!'

I watch him leave the room and, as he does so, he turns and winks at me. Later my mum and dad return with even better news.

'How would you like to come home for the weekend?'

'What?'

'Mr Peach has said you can spend the weekend at home if you like,' says Mum.

'But how will I manage?' I ask.

'Well, you get round here in your chair, so it should be okay at home. Dad or Martin can carry you upstairs.'

'Yes,' adds Dad. 'Martin and Franny could both come home for the weekend. We can all be together again.'

'Yes! Oh please! I would love to come home!'

'That's sorted then.' Mum is determined. 'We will have a wonderful time.'

The day has turned round since my dawn conversation with Steve. Now I am able to see some kind of future, even if it is very uncertain. I feel so excited about going home.

Later I go to see the Ward Six boys and tell them the news about my tests being clear. They are pleased for me and delighted to hear of my shortened stay at Christie's but there is an atmosphere of gloom.

'We'll miss you, kid!' says Barry, and I tell them I will miss them too. We have a laugh and Peter pours out some more vodka. After a while I am left alone with Barry. 'Come and see me when you get back!' he jokes and I promise I will, although I don't know if I will ever see him again. I do know that, even though the chemotherapy drugs could cure me, they are so poisonous they might also kill me – that's if the Limpet doesn't get me first. But I try not to think about that because I don't want to spoil this night. We hold hands and listen to his music. It is the first night I have been allowed to stay here so late but the nurses make an exception. By the time I get back to Ward Eight all the other patients are tucked up and sleeping.

Friday arrives too quickly. I am so looking forward to spending time at home and seeing my family again but I will miss my new friends and I am a little scared of leaving the familiar territory of the hospital. I have so many hurdles to face.

Mr Peach comes to see me early.

'Right, Little Lady, I need to see your stump. Then I need to take the stitches out of your wound.'

'I hate that word "stump", Mr Peach, don't you?'

'Mmm, yes, I do.'

'It sounds so ugly and final,' I explain. It conjures up pictures of bleeding soldiers I remember from my history books, or scenes from torture chambers.

'Well, what do you want to call it, then?' Mr Peach asks.

I think for a moment.

'Let's call it my Little Leg!'

'Okay then, much better,' he agrees 'A Little Leg for a Little Lady.'

'Do you want to see your Little Leg now?' he asks, for I have still not had the courage to look at it without the bandages on. He pauses. 'You have to at some time, you know.'

I look at him and nod, for I know I will be strong enough while he is here. He finishes unwinding the layers and layers of bandages and slowly removes the dressings to view his stitching.

'Ready?' he asks and takes my hand. I look at my Little Leg. I expected it to be ugly and horrible, but it isn't. I had pictured it as bloody and bruised but it is pink and soft and healed. Quite cute, really. My new body is not ugly, just different.

'It's very neat,' I say to him.

'Thank you. I tried my best. Why don't I leave you here for a few minutes while I go and get some stuff to take out your stitches?'

He leaves me alone with my new body and disappears. I look curiously at myself. I am changed but not mutilated. I feel sadness but no longer hatred for my own body. Maybe I am not as ugly as I assumed.

I scream as Mr Peach takes the stitches out. 'Make as much noise as you like!' he says, so I do. When he is finished he looks at me with a serious face.

'You must be very careful, Mary,' he says kindly. 'Your Little Leg is very delicate still. Don't knock it, under any circumstances.'

'What would happen if I did?'

'Well, the wound is healed but not very strong. First, it would hurt a lot, but it could also open up the wound and that would be a disaster. So just be careful – no tearing around on crutches when you get to Christie's.'

'I will be very, very careful,' I promise him.

I am tired after my ordeal and sleep for a long time. Before I know it, my family is gathering to take me home. Hellie arrives first.

'We have so many surprises planned for the weekend,' she tells me. 'I've brought you some clothes.' She hands them to me and I am delighted. They are, as all her clothes are, incredibly well-chosen. I select an outfit. I get to the bottom of the bag and pull out a new shoe.

'Hellie, you only put one shoe in,' I say, unthinkingly. She reaches over and gives me a playful hug.

'Silly! You only need one now – until you get your new leg.' Now I know why Mum sent Hellie early; she never makes a big deal out of it. I stare at her, wondering how I feel, and then I decide it has a funny side and I laugh. She laughs, too.

'How can you forget you have only one leg, Mary?'

Hellie helps me pack. We fill several large bags with cards and presents. The cards have covered most of the walls for the last few weeks and there are literally hundreds. Mum and Dad return with presents for the nurses and Dr Jimmy. For the first time in three weeks I don outdoor clothes. Hellie helps me dress my leg with a stocking and my lonely shoe. There are so many new things to face.

'Are you okay, Sis?'

'Just thinking.'

'What about? Your leg?' I nod and sigh. 'Look at it this way – you only have to buy half as many stockings!' she jokes and we both fall about laughing. Dr Jimmy comes into the room.

'What's all the noise in here?' He pretends to be cross at us. 'I've come to say goodbye and thank you for the chocolates.'

'That's okay, Jimmy. Thanks for looking after me.'

Mr Peach rushes in. 'You be good at Christie's, now,' he tells me, 'and I'll see you when you get back, by which time I hope we can sort you out with an artificial leg.'

'Fantastic! I can't wait!'

'I'm very proud of you, Little Lady. You have been remarkably brave. I won't forget the things you've taught me.'

'Me? Taught you?'

'Well, I know now that some words are difficult for my patients. That's a useful lesson for me.'

I bask in his compliments and I am determined that, if I get through my treatment, I will pass my exams so I can come back and tell him. We give each other a big hug and I feel a sense of loss as he leaves.

'Ready?' asks Hellie when she has done my make-up and hair for me.

'You bet. Let's get out of here.'

I reach for my blanket but Hellie snatches it away.

'No, you're not having that. You don't need it. It makes you look like a granny. You are beautiful as you are.'

'People will stare at me, though,' I complain.

'Then I will stare back. That's before I run them over with the wheel-chair!'

'I can't wait for Franny to arrive too!' I say. 'It will be great for us to be three again.'

'Well, I have an idea,' Hellie says as she pushes me briskly out of the ward. 'From now on we will all three of us share legs. That makes one point something each!'

'Bye-bye, Ward Eight!' we shout together.

Dad is waiting with the car at the front of the hospital. He straps me in the front and speaks to Hellie.

'You must hold Mary's shoulders from behind so she doesn't over-balance when I go round corners.'

I hold tightly to the car seat, for I am indeed unbalanced. He drives very slowly and, by the time we get home, I feel like a cripple. I am exhausted and I haven't done anything. Mum has cooked a special dinner for me but, having eaten it, I am ready for bed. I hear the door banging and the loud voice of my older brother. He has come home from university to see me.

'Where's my little sister?' I hear him shout. He comes bounding in. 'You look great!' he says to me and doesn't even look at my wheelchair. 'Have a present from the gang at uni!' and he fastens a delicate gold bracelet around my wrist.

'It's beautiful,' I say and admire it. He has made me feel special and worthy.

'Okay, so it's up the stairs, is it?' and he scoops me up in his arms and climbs the stairs two at a time. Hellie comes up to our pretty room, too, and sits on the bed with me.

'I'll stay with you, Mary,' she says and strokes my hair. 'When you wake up in the morning, Franny will be here too.' She kisses me gently and lies down beside me. I feel safe and loved.

I sleep heavily and when I wake it is light and the room is empty. It must be quite late in the morning. I hear voices chattering downstairs and recognize Franny's laughter. I call down the stairs as loudly as I can. My two sisters run up to see me and we all have a huge hug.

'Oh, it's so good to be back here with you both,' I say. 'What shall we do today?'

'We are all going out for lunch later on – somewhere really smart!'

'This afternoon we've arranged for some of your friends to come over.'

'Perhaps this morning we can go out for a walk.' I want to get out in the fresh air again. I have been deprived of the outside world. My sisters pass me my clothes. Undressed, I am a little self-conscious these days.

'Mary, you are so thin,' Hellie notices. 'I must tell Mum you need feeding up.'

Franny hunts around the room for her camera and then calls my brother to carry me downstairs again. Everything seems so difficult now. I think back to how easy it used to be to run downstairs two at a time. Now getting downstairs is a huge performance.

'I want some pictures of you two to take back to college with me,' Franny explains as she pushes my wheelchair up to the park.

Even though it is still January, it is mild with a hint of spring in the air. I shiver, though, after only a few minutes. My body has been in a warm hospital for so long I have forgotten what it's like to feel cold. I look at the snowdrops and the bulbs pushing through the soil and wonder to myself whether I will ever see them flower. I have started to count in days and weeks. I have begun to set myself little goals to aim for. I decide to set myself one now. Next weekend the snowdrops will just about be flowering so that will be my goal – to come here and see the snowdrops. At the park we have fun and I enjoy myself but I am also aware that everything now is tinged with sadness. Nothing is the same and never will be. My sisters and I have been up here so often, running and jumping and practising our gymnastics. I will never do these things again. But I am here. I am alive. I shudder as I think back to Thursday morning and my trip down the long corridor. Franny sees me shiver.

'Time to get you home,' she says. 'But first a photo!' She asks a passing dog-walker to picture the three of us. He looks at me sympathetically. I see the look of pity in his eyes as my sisters help me stand. It suddenly strikes me, as he is snapping away, that these may be the last photos of us three girls together. I realize now why Franny wanted to bring her camera. Aim for the snowdrops, I tell myself. Then aim for the daffodils. For after the winter comes springtime and new life.

At lunchtime my dad takes us all out for a treat. We have a wonderful time at the restaurant. The whole family is together again. I watch my mum and dad looking at us all and I realize they are thinking the same as Franny. They are wondering how many more times we shall all be together like this. I sit between my two sisters. I spend a lot of time talking to Martin and telling him about God helping me through my illness. I thought that being strong in all this would bring him back to God, but it has had the opposite effect. He hates God now for allowing it to happen. He is angry, he says, at what I have gone through. Why didn't God intervene and rescue you, he asks me, and I don't know how to answer. Why should you have to suffer this way, he says. My little brother, Adrian, is silent. He doesn't say a word. He won't speak to my dad and barely looks at my mum. It seems to me he blames them for making the decision to allow the operation. He thinks it is their fault that I have lost my leg.

With a shock I realize our entire family has been touched by my illness. I see now that we all have cancer one way or another. We all feel grief, anger and guilt. We all feel pain and uncertainty. We are all very scared.

Sunday morning arrives and with it the usual church routine. Because I am home the entire family goes to Mass, even Martin, but he sits there stony-faced. I sit in my wheelchair at the side of the hard church bench, feeling conspicuous and on display. At the end of Mass a large crowd of well-wishers gathers around me. Lots of people come over and clasp my hand. 'You're so brave!' they all say to me and I feel bewildered at their choice of words. They all smile sweetly and treat me like some sort of saint. I am not brave at all. I just don't have a choice. If there was an easier way I would take it – although I now know I am not yet ready for suicide. After a while I tire of the trite platitudes and ask my sisters to take me home.

Franny has a train to catch after lunch and I cry as she leaves. She promises to write and come over and see me in Christie's. Hellie gets stuck into her homework and Adrian heads off to practise his music. Soon Martin has to return as well.

'See you in Manchester, Sis,' he promises. The house is all too quiet. I potter around in my wheelchair, feeling gloomy.

Later, I am sent an invitation to join the God Squad for an Italian meal. Except for pizzas, I have never had Italian food before. I am told I must order mushrooms and garlic bread.

As I prepare to set off, I think how strange it is – there are so many things I have never done. I have never eaten garlic bread before. I've never been abroad. I've never made love with anybody and I'll never

47

wear a beautiful white wedding dress. I've never drunk red wine in a grown-up restaurant. I haven't seen medical school. I might not even make it to my A levels. And, do you know, I have never held a sweet newborn baby. Let alone had my own child which will never, ever be. And that makes me so unhappy.

I make a mental list of all the things I would like to do. I start to imagine medical school. I remember stories Dr Jimmy told me to make me laugh. It must be such fun, apart from dissecting bodies.

The restaurant is dark and cosy. I have never been anywhere like it before. There are bright candles in bottles, and guitar music plays in the background. Waiters appear carrying delicious creations, and one rushes over. He rearranges the tables and fits us in a corner. I order mushrooms, garlic bread and cannelloni. We drink red wine and feel very grown-up. The meal arrives and I taste it.

'It's delicious!' I say, and everyone laughs. We have a good time; the food is wonderful, the waiter tops up our glasses and we all joke and laugh about school. The evening rushes by and, before I know it, we reach our curfew. But, back home, I lie in my bed dreading what lies ahead at Christie's. I want time to stop. I cuddle up to my sister. She stirs in her sleep and flings her arm protectively around me.

I think back to my happiest moment with my sisters when we all ran hand in hand down a Scottish mountain, our cheeks red and our hair flying loose. We sat on a huge boulder overlooking a loch on the last family holiday before I got sick. I remember seeing the moon, large and pale, reflected in the water and thinking how much beauty was in the world. Now I have seen another side of life. I recall that I shivered, for it was getting cold and late by the lake, but none of us wanted to forsake the moment so my big sister wrapped her cardigan around my shoulders and gave me a hug. We sang, my sisters and I, 'Over the sea to Skye'. I hum it under my breath. I feel a desolate sadness.

'Over the sea to anywhere,' I whisper, 'but not here, please, not here.'

Hellie shakes me awake in the morning. She is already in her school uniform. Blackness hits me immediately. Christie's beckons.

'I'll see you Friday. Be brave for me.'

I am unable to speak, fighting back tears. She wipes my eyes.

'You'll be okay.'

'Oh, Hellie,' I sob loudly and she holds me and rocks me. The cancer, the pain, the disability, the fear and confusion, I want it all to end.

'Shh. I'll always be there for you. Even if I'm not physically there. I'll be with you in spirit. And Franny too. Okay? Just think of us holding your hands.'

I wipe my eyes and whisper: 'Yes, that's what I'll think of.'

'Think of our special times together. All the wonderful things we have done together. Think of those things when you feel alone. We'll do those things again, I promise.'

Mid-morning, two jolly ambulancemen lift me onto a stretcher and tuck a blanket around me.

'Try to sleep,' one of them advises. Mum and Dad follow in their car.

Soon we arrive at Christie's. I am instantly disappointed. I imagined a small friendly place. This is a huge tower block with rows of impersonal windows. I am taken to a busy clinic area where Mum and Dad meet me. There are no friendly faces or people who stop and say hello to my dad. I feel small and insignificant. We are called in to see Dr Pearson after a long wait during which I fall asleep. She examines me and then talks to my mum and dad, but not to me. She is brusque and businesslike and barks out her questions. I feel completely ignored. There are no smiles or small talk here.

'You are going to Ward Two,' my parents tell me after a separate consultation with the doctor. 'It's an adult ward. Dr Pearson couldn't decide whether to put you on the children's or the adults' ward, but we thought you might prefer to be quieter if you wanted to study or something.'

The corridors are long with signs and notices for 'Radiotherapy' and 'Isotope Room' and one that I recognize for a CT scanner. At Ward Two a nurse in a dark blue sister's uniform comes out to meet us.

'Hello, Mary!' she greets me with a broad smile. 'I'm Sister Anna. We have been looking forward to meeting you. We've heard a lot about you.'

She is tiny and very thin and has long blonde hair. She has a lovely smile and I feel more at ease.

'This is Vera. She'll show you round the ward.'

A very fat nurse bustles over to me with a wheelchair. She helps me into it and turns to my mum and dad. 'Do you want to go now? I'll help Mary unpack.'

My parents haven't said much since the interview with Dr Pearson and they seem upset again.

They give me hugs and leave me with Vera who helps me take in my new surroundings. This place will be my temporary home for several months. I spot some strange yellow signs posted round several of the beds. 'Danger! Radiation hazard!' There is a black symbol on the sign, too, which I recognize from an experiment we did in physics. It means that something is radioactive.

'What's the sign for?' I ask Vera.

'The yellow sign indicates that the patient has a radioactive implant inside their body. It would be dangerous to go too near. Whenever you see those signs, you must keep away from the bed.'

I have a distant memory. I am sure I have seen the sign a long time ago, even before my physics lessons. I rack my brain and try to think when it was. I remember I was very small, maybe only five or six … Martin was with me. We were playing – somewhere dark and danger-ous but I'm not sure where.

Although Ward Two is different from Ward Eight at the Victoria, it isn't too bad. The beds are all lined up on either side of the long narrow ward and all have names. Vera stops at an empty one. It is called the Edith Cavell bed.

'Here you are, this is Edith!' she jokes. She lifts me out of the chair onto the bed and starts unpacking. All the women on the ward are old, apart from one other girl and me. She seems about my age and I notice she walks with a limp.

'Who's that?' I ask curiously.

'That's Debbie. She's had a bone tumour. She has an artificial leg.'

'What? I couldn't even tell. When did she get hers?'

'Ages ago. Two years, I think.'

'Oh. I don't understand. Why is she here, then?'

Vera doesn't answer at first. Then, 'She has come back for some check-ups and things.'

'Maybe I could ask her about legs and that kind of stuff?'

'Yes, but I'll warn you, she doesn't like talking about it much.'

Vera unpacks my Bible and some prayer books. 'You believe in God, then?'

'Oh yes, definitely. He is going to heal me, you know. I might not need the chemotherapy.'

'Listen to this girl,' Vera says loudly, to the ward in general. 'Isn't she brave?'

'What is wrong with you, then?' asks one of the ladies. 'What have you got?'

'I haven't got anything now. I'm better. I'm just here to have chemotherapy. God has healed me, you see.'

The lady looks puzzled and Vera is silent. I can see I'll have my work cut out to teach them about miracles.

After a couple of hours I am bored. Nothing happens here. There is no Ward Six to visit and no Dr Jimmy to make a fuss of me. Lots of the ladies have bits of their bodies missing. One lady has a breast missing and looks all lopsided. She covers her top half with shawls. I think it must be really awful and wonder if they give you an artificial breast and what she will do about wearing a bra. Every time I look at her she looks away from me. Maybe she is embarrassed about me seeing her. It doesn't dawn on me until later that maybe she thinks I am lopsided too. Another lady talks about cancer all the time. She has had a bowel tumour and has a bag on her tummy. It must be horribly messy and smelly. I tell her I want to be a doctor which is a big mistake because she tells me horror stories about all the operations she and her friends have undergone. She points to the lady in the next bed and tells me she only has half a tongue. She tells the lady to show me and the lady sticks her tongue out. It looks so ugly and strange.

Another lady is bald. In fact, lots of the ladies are bald and, from time to time, they take off their wigs to brush them or scratch their heads. I wondered what it would look like and now I know. I sort of thought that everybody would be wearing long blonde wigs and that kind of thing but, no, she is sitting there with her head as bald as an egg. She looks weird. I don't want to look weird. I am scared of my hair falling out. It might sound stupid but in some ways it is more scary than cancer. I spend a lot of time making my hair look nice. It is one of my better points – that and my eyes. I don't really feel confident about my appearance. I think I'm too skinny and my boobs are too small. I can't stand my freckles either. But my hair is lovely, wavy and soft. I had nice legs too but now I can't have nice legs. I can only have a nice leg and that's weird, too. So now I will be even weirder with no hair. It is so freaky, this place. People walking around with strange bodies – bits missing and lopsided and things like that. It's like seeing aliens off *Star Trek* and now I'm one of them. And I don't want to be.

I wheel into the day room and sit on my own for a while. I feel a rising panic. I can't stay here; it is awful. I am surrounded by sickness and old age. There is an atmosphere of imminent death and gloom. I look out of the window and see the bare trees. All these ladies seem to be very sick, and it dawns on me that maybe I am, too. Cancer means death and destruction. It is all around me, the inevitable decay. I feel so lonely and desperate.

The door opens and Vera comes in. She sits beside me and smiles.

'What are you thinking about?'

'I guess I feel scared.'

'My best friend was ill in here. She had treatment. That's why I nurse here.'

'What happened to her?'

'She's fine now. She fought it. That's what you have to do. Fight. Don't give up. Ignore the other ladies. It's how they cope, talking about their illnesses, but you're too young for that.'

'But there's nothing to do.'

'Well, get your mum to bring your school books in. There's no reason why you can't read when it's quiet.'

'Is there a library?'

'No, but there is a chapel and it's very quiet up there.'

She agrees to take me after lunch. I like her. She is a kind and motherly person with a smile always on her face. We sit next to each other in the chapel and talk.

'My friend believes in God, too,' Vera whispers. 'She says that her faith has got her through.'

'Is she a Catholic?' I ask.

'No, I don't think so. But it doesn't matter, does it? I must introduce you to Irene as well. She's the staff nurse on the ward. She is also a Christian. Her faith is very strong.'

The chapel is beautiful and so peaceful. It is dark and cool. It seems a long way from the wards and is very quiet. I notice it is not Catholic. It doesn't seem to make any difference except there aren't any statues of Our Lady. A large tapestry picture of the Last Supper hangs on the wall with Jesus breaking bread. I try to work out which figure is Judas. He must be the one with the evil smile.

'You must be cold and tired,' interrupts Vera. 'Let's get you back.'

The doctor arrives. I call him Dr Tan-Shoes. He doesn't tell me his name. He looks briefly in my direction and starts to read my notes. He doesn't talk to me at all. Then he comes up and takes my arms without explanation. I pull them away.

'What are you doing?'

'Veins. I'm looking for veins.' He continues his search and sighs. 'Your veins are bad. That will be a problem.'

I begin to worry. What does he mean?

'When does my chemotherapy start? Today?'

'No. Next week.' I am surprised and ask him why.

'Tests. We need to do more tests.' He is walking away as he says it. I feel really angry because he won't explain things to me.

'But I've had loads of tests.'

'We need to repeat them.'

I sit there and simmer with anger. What a waste of time, I think, when I could be home.

The week is long and dull. The tests are repeated, exactly as before, only this time nobody comes to tell me the results. I find them out from my parents when they visit. I am grumpy and depressed the whole week. I lie on the bed and try to concentrate on reading, but it is difficult. The only breaks in the routine are mealtimes. I get to know the nurses and the physio. She brings a set of crutches and helps me use them. Her manner is also sharp and matter-of-fact.

'We can't have you in a wheelchair all the time. You'll become weak and you won't be able to manage an artificial leg.'

'Well, how will I get around?'

'On crutches. You've got arms.' She makes me do exercises every day and soon I am worn out with her pummelling. In the end she takes away my wheelchair and leaves me with only the crutches. I hate them because I can't hide the fact that I am minus a leg and I feel self-conscious and embarrassed.

By Thursday I am all packed up, ready to go home and determined I am not coming back. The chemotherapy will have to go and God will just have to do a miracle without it. I ask myself how I can possibly tell people about God here, where nothing happens.

I am lying on my bed in a bad mood when a nurse walks up to me. She is short and plump.

'Hi, Mary. I'm Irene. Vera told me you're a Christian, too.' I sit up quickly. This seems better.

I tell her: 'I've been waiting to meet you. I don't know why God has brought me here. There is absolutely nothing I can do for Him here. I've decided not to come back next week.'

'That's a real shame because there are some books I think you will really enjoy about people who have been through difficult times. I was thinking they would help you.'

'Well, I bet they haven't been through anything as awful as this.' I am really feeling sorry for myself now.

'One is about a girl called Joni who breaks her neck but goes on to become a painter. And one is about Nicky Cruz, who is a drug addict and a gang member who becomes a preacher. Sounds pretty awful to me.'

'I'm sick of people going on about God and how He can get me through. It's just a cop-out.'

Irene looks at me and laughs. 'Well, do you have any other option? You're not doing so good on your own, are you?'

'No, I'm not really,' I have to admit. 'I'll give it one more try.'

So I went home for the weekend. I had a lovely time and the snowdrops had bloomed – Hellie took me up to the park to see them. Now I am back. My tests are finished and my chemotherapy starts tomorrow. Irene has brought in the books for me and I'm saving them for when my treatment starts.

Dr Pearson came to see me this morning. She explained about the chemotherapy. I asked her about my hair. She said it will all fall out in a few weeks. I'm praying it won't. I asked Dr Pearson about being infertile and she looked at me as if I was crazy. She said: 'One step at a time.'

But it is important to me. If God is going to heal me, and I live, I want to have children. That's if anyone will ever love me. I guess that someone would have to be different and special to be able to love me now. I started to cry, and one of the ladies went to get Irene and she came and had a chat. She is a very gentle person. She said Jesus can help me through all the bad times and I will be very close to Him because of suffering like this. She said: 'Think of Him as your best friend.' She is really helping me to understand God.

As the day goes by I feel more and more frightened about starting the chemotherapy. Debbie is now having some and she keeps being very sick. The drugs go into the veins through a drip and I'm scared because drips hurt a lot. I don't understand why Debbie is having more chemotherapy so long after her operation. The nurses won't let me go and talk to her. They say she needs to rest. She looks very ill – thin and pale. I'm thinking maybe she has got secondaries or something and that scares me too.

Vera sees me looking worried and comes over. 'How about having a lovely bath, getting your nightdress on ready for your drip later, and then I will take you up to the chapel?'

She helps me into my nightclothes and walks me up to the chapel. I am pretty good on my crutches now and when we get there she suggests I might like some time alone. I want to pray.

She leaves me alone in the cool silence. Nobody comes up here, ever. Once I saw the hospital chaplain and he said hello but, apart from that, only I come up here with my books and my Bible. I am reading the Psalms. Irene said they were good things to read in hard times. So I do as she told me and ask God to speak to me through His word and then I open the Bible at Psalm 6 and begin to read. I'm sure God will tell me something really important with my treatment starting tomorrow.

I read words that do not fit the picture: 'O Lord, do not rebuke me in your anger ...'

Why is He angry? Is it because it is all my fault?

'... or discipline me in your wrath.'

Discipline? Oh no – that must be my illness, maybe even secondaries. I knew it was a punishment.

'Be merciful to me ...'

But why do I need mercy? Is it because I'm a bad person?

'O Lord heal me, for my bones are in agony.'

That's me! It's talking about me. My bones are in agony. Of course. Why didn't I see? The cancer is a punishment for my sin and for the bad things I've done in my life. Maybe I will get secondaries and then I will die.

I am crying and sobbing, the tears flowing steadily and easily down my cheeks.

I know the cancer can kill me – and even if the cancer doesn't then the drugs might. They will poison my body, cell by cell. First they will poison my scalp and my hair will fall out, leaving me a bald and sexless freak. Then my ovaries will die, robbing me of the beautiful children I have always longed for. Then, maybe then, the bad cells left by the Limpet will be poisoned. They might be killed; they might not. If they aren't poisoned then I will certainly die. 'Death', a word I never used until recently, has now entered my vocabulary and is used every day of my life. I feel I can't escape from its shadow. I dwell constantly in reach of its beckoning hand. I do not know how to die. I do not know what awaits me beyond the grave. What if I am facing an eternity in hell?

Maybe by making some painful sacrifice I can make it up to God. I cling onto the bench and kneel carefully and painstakingly on my one good knee, leaning the weight of my body over the bench. It hurts as the hard wood digs into my breasts and ribs. I should be punished. I deserve it all; the cancer, the amputation, the ugly and deformed body. The tears pour down my cheeks and run on to the bench, then cascade to the polished floor.

I look accusingly at the picture on the wall. I see the figures of Jesus and the apostles breaking bread together.

'Why me? Why me?' I sob, but the figure of Jesus is serenely aloof.

'Don't just sit there looking holy,' I yell in my mind with all the anger I am capable of.

Suddenly something inside me breaks. My mind begins to fracture and unravel. The images from the picture blur behind my tears and the figures seem to come alive. My mind leaves the chapel and I am in the upper room, sharing a passover meal. I sit down between two figures. On my right is Jesus. He is dressed in white and has a sad smile on his face. His eyes are downcast. He is crying and somehow I feel cheated. Jesus is not meant to cry. Then I see why. His hands are wounded and covered in blood. I recoil in horror at the sight. Jesus is holding a chalice full of ruby wine which catches the candlelight. He passes it to me and solemnly I lift it to my lips. I take a sip and, as I taste the metallic tang of blood, I drop the chalice and it hits the ground, smashing into millions of tiny pieces. There is blood everywhere now.

'It's broken!' I cry, and Jesus looks down. He spots the hideous, empty space where my leg no longer is. I hear Him draw breath sharply and He shakes His head disbelievingly.

'What happened to your leg?' He asks.

'They took it away. It was bad. The miracle didn't work, you see.'

Suddenly, another figure leans over my shoulder. I peer up at him and know it must be Judas because he is carrying a bag with coins in it. I hear the chink of metal on metal.

'It must have been your fault, then,' says Judas. 'What did you do wrong?'

'Nothing,' I cry. 'I don't think I did anything wrong. I don't know why it didn't work. Anyway,' I ask Jesus between sobs, 'what happened to Your hands?'

'Oh, they crucified Him,' interrupts Judas. 'I betrayed Him.' He throws his head back in mocking laughter and, as he does so, I glimpse a dark ring around his neck.

'What is that mark – like a bruise?'

Judas is silent; he looks shiftily around for a way of escape but he cannot get out of the picture.

'Tell her, Judas. Tell her you could no longer live with yourself. Tell her you hanged yourself from a tree.'

'How did he betray You?' I ask but, before He can answer, my mind leaves the scene and returns to my head. I am in the chapel again, shivering and trembling.

But in my moment of darkest fear I find courage. I recall the voice I heard when I wanted to kill myself and realize now it was the voice of Judas. I make a vow and, as I speak it to the Limpet, I know it to be true. I will survive, if only to tell the tale. Words flood into my mind from a power greater than my frail human spirit: 'I shall not die! I shall not die; but I shall live!'

Somehow I make my way back to the ward knowing that, by my own strength or by divine miracle, I must overcome death.

5

The nightmare was terrible. I was so scared. It was horrific. I woke up sweating and drenched, my heart racing. I had wet myself. All I could hear was the sound of blood pumping in my ears and breath rasping in my chest. Maybe it was because of the chemotherapy and the drip or maybe it was because of my experience in the chapel. I'm not sure.

I saw a pack of hungry dogs. They were huge and ferocious. Their fur was a mixture of tan and black. One was faster and bigger than the others. His muscles were lean and strong. His teeth were white and hard and from his mouth drooled spit. The metal spikes on his collar shone as they caught the moonlight. I tried to run and at first it felt good. I was laughing with the ease of out-running the pack. But then I fell, down, down a long, long way and the dog was upon me. The laugh became a scream. His teeth ripped into the soft muscles of my left thigh and I felt agonizing pain and the crunch of splintering bone as his canines met and easily split my limb. The blood spurted skyward and the dog picked up my severed leg and shook it in his mouth. I could see his tongue relishing the taste of my blood. I struggled to roll over and push the killer away. But before I knew it his teeth were at my neck, ready to execute me. I should look my killer in the eye, I thought, in the courage and the despair of my final moment, and so I looked into the eyes of a murderer. I do not understand.

Yesterday Dr Tan-Shoes came to put my drip in. That was awful too. He walked up to me and nodded, carrying a shiny metal dish shaped like a bean. In it were lots of needles with plastic blobs on them, all different colours: pink and blue and green. He chose a green one. It seemed bigger than the other needles. They looked pretty sitting in the dish and I thought maybe it would not be too bad. Irene had already brought a pole with a bag of salt water hanging on it to attach to the needle. Dr Tan-Shoes held my arm and put a tight band around it to make my veins fill up. He started to shake his head and made tutting noises. Then he got the needle and stuck it in my arm and I jumped in the bed because it hurt so much. I drew my arm back and he got really cross and said the vein had popped. Blood was running all down my arm. He tried again and again but he just couldn't get the needle in my vein and he kept getting more and more impatient. I got scared and it was hurting me so much and then I cried, but he didn't say anything. He just kept sticking the needle in my arm. I was shaking by the end of it and there was blood everywhere, all over my bedspread. It must be very difficult to put a drip in. Then he attached the needle to the bag of fluid and went. The nurses gave me lots of tablets to help my kidneys work properly and told me the chemotherapy would start next day.

This morning, Irene came to make my bed and noticed it was all wet from my nightmare. I told her I spilt the bedpan. She washed and changed me, for I am stuck here now, chained to the bed by my drip.

'You look tired, Mary,' she said to me. 'Didn't you get any sleep?'

'Not much.' I didn't sleep after the nightmare – I was too scared.

'Are you worrying about starting the drugs? What are you thinking about, Mary?'

'I was wondering if God gets angry with people. You know, for bad things they have done.'

'No, Mary. God isn't like that. He loves you – especially now you are going through pain.'

I fixed my plaster saint smile to my face and nodded in agreement. But inside I am black and hopeless.

Dr Tan-Shoes appears with a drip bag containing a bright yellow fluid. It looks so cheerful – but it is deadly poison.

'What is that?' I ask him.

'Methotrexate,' he says. I file the name away to ask my dad about it tomorrow when he visits me.

He picks up a syringe with something in it and injects it into a little hole underneath the green blob on the needle.

'And that one?'

'Vincristine.' He selects another, much bigger, syringe.

'So what is that one for?' I am trying really hard to be nice to him to make up for my veins being so bad. Maybe then he will like me, too.

'To stop you being sick.'

'And my hair …?'

He starts to walk away and, as he does, throws back a comment: 'It will fall out now.'

I stare at the bedcover and the pattern blurs as tears well up in my eyes and spill onto my nightdress. I am crying because it seems as if my hair can be thrown away as casually as his remark. My hair is more precious than that. I am only seventeen and my hair is so pretty. I have been growing it. The lady in the bed opposite – the one with the tummy bag – is cross.

'He shouldn't tell you like that!' she says, and storms up the ward to find Irene who comes and sits on the bed and gives me a hug. I am so tired of losing all that I have. It is as if my body doesn't belong to me any more.

I watch the yellow drug dripping into my vein and wait anxiously to see how I feel. It advances in a bright wave down the tube and I can see it entering my body. It doesn't take long. Soon I begin to heave and retch and the covers are now soaked in blood and tears and vomit. And this is how it is for the next two days. My body is racked with spasm after spasm and heaves with the strain of emptying itself of yellow poison. The hours pass in a haze and I am only vaguely aware of the morning becoming afternoon. Nurses come and go, bringing me snacks and drinks which lie untouched. Mum visits me and talks but it is like living in twilight and when she is gone I do not know if she was ever really there. Then it is night and I drift in and out of the nightmare, the same awful nightmare, only this time I know the ending and I am even more scared.

I wake and hear the rasping breath of the lady in the next bed. She is frail and old. She has been very ill and cannot even speak. I hear the noise of her gasping and her chest rattling as my own breathless fears subside. It sounds as if her every breath is an effort. I listen to her drowning for several hours. Sometimes she moans softly in pain. And sometimes she whispers the name of a man, 'Jack'. Nobody comes to sit by her, for it is late and she is so old. The drowning noise gets worse and I call, hesitantly, for a nurse – not knowing whether I should, but all the other ladies are asleep. The nurses cannot hear me and no-one comes to her. Suddenly, there is silence. I wait for the next breath but it doesn't come. I hold my breath too. When I can no longer resist the urge to gulp in a huge lungful of air, I listen again. The noises are definitely gone. She is no longer breathing. Why has she stopped breathing, I wonder, and I wait for something to happen but the silence goes on.

And then I realize. She is dead. I have heard the old lady die. She has died of cancer.

I quell an overwhelming desire to scream and scream. I have never heard death before. The other ladies still sleep. I call again for a nurse and think maybe I should have done something before to help. Maybe I should have called louder and then she would not have died. Perhaps the nurses will be angry I did not call louder to summon assistance. I feel a rising sense of panic. So I lie quietly in my bed, pretending to be asleep, in case it turns out to be my fault.

A short time later I hear the nurses approach her.

'Ah, she has gone at last,' one whispers to the other.

'It's for the best,' the other says and I hear them rustling about the bedside and drawing the curtains. I turn over and weep softly into my pillow and taste the salt of my tears. I am in a ward where people are dying and old and mutilated. I am a part of it and I do not want to be. I want to be young and pretty and back to how I was. If I can't have that, then I don't want anything.

I hear the voice of Judas again in my mind, clear and insistent.

'You don't want to die like that, do you?'

'Like what?'

'Alone and in pain and drowning.'

'But it's wrong. Suicide is wrong. I would go to hell.'

'You're dying anyway. Why do you think you're here?'

And the voice is right. This is a hopeless place. All the ladies are ill and one of them just died, right here in the next bed. It could be me next. So I might as well kill myself the way I choose rather than die like that old lady. I want to die at home, not here on my own in a lonely and desperate place.

'How can I do it? I'm chained to my bed. I can't even move.'

But I begin to think of a way. I plan it all out. I feel calmer, knowing I can make the decision to kill myself. At least I won't have to guess any more. I curl up and sleep the sleep of exhaustion.

Next day the yellow drug is finished. Dr Tan-Shoes comes to my bedside and takes away the empty bag and replaces it with salt water. After a few hours the vomiting stops and, although I am tired, I feel a little better. I sit up and eat something and then Irene comes and gives me a bed-bath.

Mum and Dad visit later in the afternoon. They greet me with hugs and a bag full of cards and presents from friends and relatives. My dad still looks strained and anxious but my mum seems to have become the strong one now. I see she is the glue which holds the family together.

I tell my dad about the drip not going in and he looks at the bruises on my arms. He seems upset and rushes off to talk to Sister and then I am worried in case Dr Tan-Shoes dislikes me even more. Our afternoon together passes so quickly. I feel lonely when they wave goodbye and cry again when they leave.

I lie on my bed, resting, watching the tiny drops of salt water drip into my blood, helping my body to recover, and I begin to think about death again. The thoughts just pop into my head, especially when I am alone. They are black and frightening. My mind is full of worry and fear. I am glad when Vera comes over and sits on my bed.

'Missing Mum and Dad?' she asks. 'Well, home tomorrow for the weekend. We will give you all your tablets to take home with you and then you come back on Monday to have your blood checked before starting the next dose of chemotherapy.'

'What tablets do I take home, then?'

'Your painkillers, some sleeping tablets, all the antidotes to the chemotherapy and plenty of anti-sickness tablets, too. Are you still getting bad pain?'

In truth, my pain is easing now.

'Yes, it is still pretty awful,' I say innocently.

'Okay, we'll get you something good and strong. How about your sleep?'

I have hardly slept a wink, even with the sleeping tablets, so hoarding them and not taking them will not make much difference.

'Yes, I'll need sleeping tablets too – and lots of pills for sickness.'

Vera bustles off to sort them out for me. If I save them and hide them, in a few weeks I will have plenty. Painkillers and sleeping tablets would be a good way. It wouldn't hurt. I would just get sleepier and sleepier. I might even have enough time to ask God to forgive me. I feel elated when Vera comes over with a sealed brown envelope. I have found an escape route.

After supper I doze with the curtains drawn around me. I feel as if I want to shut the rest of the world out of the little bit of space that belongs to me. I stare at the frayed curtains and count the squares on the patterned and worn material. I reach for the envelope and count the tablets. There are about twenty strong painkillers and four sleeping tablets. It should take about three weeks until I have enough, I guess, and I hide them beneath my schoolfriends' letters in my bedside drawer.

Thursday arrives and I am excited. I am going home today! Dr Tan-Shoes arrives and takes down the dreaded drip and I am free to go where I want again. I soak in a deep hot bath and plan the weekend ahead. I shampoo my hair slowly and carefully, tugging at it to see if it is dying yet, but it seems to be all there still. I spend a long time drying my hair and savouring the feeling of running my hands through the long, soft strands. I dress in my outdoor clothes for the first time in days and wait for my dad to arrive to take me home.

The journey from Manchester is long and tiring and I feel sick most of the way but it is so good to be with my family again. Hellie meets me joyfully at the door.

'I have such a weekend planned for you!' she tells me as she wheels me to the safe refuge of our bedroom and squeezes my hands. 'You'll never be alone with your sisters beside you. We will always be together.'

I look into her beautiful green eyes and think again about what I am contemplating. To take my own life would be taking part of hers away, too. I decide I will carry on saving the tablets but give things a few more weeks. I am eighteen soon; I will live until my birthday and then decide.

Hellie is allowed to take the day off school on Friday as a special treat. She and Mum are taking me into town in my wheelchair. It is the first time I have been out in a public place since Boxing Day and I feel awkward and self-conscious. Hellie allows me to cover my leg with a blanket and quickly takes control. She pushes me briskly through the crowds, telling me all the school gossip. We enter a fashionable shop and a middle-aged assistant approaches and asks if we need any help.

'We need hats and things to cover up my sister's head when her hair falls out,' she explains quite calmly and naturally. I feel so proud of her and sit quietly, allowing my brave sister to do the talking.

'And what do you think your sister would like?' the bemused assistant asks politely.

'Well, you could always try asking her!' My sister can be very outspoken.

The lady asks me a few questions and points to a corner of the shop. A group of young girls is gathered there and I feel my heart sink. I am conspicuous and different. They stare at me and one of them whispers to her friend, who stares even more. I feel myself blushing and wonder if I am about to cry. Hellie rams the wheelchair into their ankles and they jump aside, rubbing their bruises. My sister smiles sweetly.

'I'm so sorry,' she says to them. 'You obviously didn't see us here. You were too busy staring!' She fixes them with an angry look and I try to restrain my laughter.

We return home loaded with shopping and I am exhausted. I am so tired that I sleep for the remainder of the afternoon, waking briefly only for supper. Hellie comes up to bed early and pushes the two matching beds together and I fall asleep in her comforting arms.

In the early hours of the morning the dogs enter my dreams once more. Again I see the beasts bearing down on me, the sweating skins and the wide staring eyes. I can smell the cloying blood and see the flecks of foam on the jaws of the biggest one as he plunges towards my neck. I awake screaming and struggling in my sister's arms. It takes a few moments before I realize where I am and my breath slows to the same steady pace as hers.

'Shh, Mary,' she soothes. 'You were dreaming. You must have had a nightmare. You punched me in the face and screamed at me to get off!'

'Oh no, I'm so sorry. It was so scary this time.'

'What were you dreaming about?'

'Dogs, I was dreaming about dogs. They were attacking me and tearing my leg off.'

'So who were you screaming at to get off you?'

'Dr Tan-Shoes.'

'Yes, well, I'm not surprised,' she says. 'Try to sleep now.' She holds me tightly and sings hymns to me until I fall asleep.

That evening I am collected and my wheelchair is packed into a car taking me to Tiggi's, a restaurant in St Anne's, where I will meet the God Squad and get to eat some more garlic bread.

My dad hands over a large plastic container. Oh no! I am embarrassed and turn bright red and feel hot. It is a bottle for my urine. I have to collect it because of the chemo so the hospital can check my kidneys. The drugs are so strong and poisonous they could cause them to fail. So the big bottle goes everywhere with me. It is already half-full of bright yellow liquid. Now it sits on the back seat and I wish the ground would swallow me up.

A large crowd of my friends has gathered at the restaurant. I hide the bottle under my rug and we all take our places. The meal is very

64

pleasant but I look out of the window and wish myself far, far away from all that has become my life – the ugly wheelchair, the curious stares, the horrid rug hiding the plastic bottle. I want to hide, too, in a safe, warm place and be normal again like my friends and sisters. I want to sit on a proper chair and wear pretty pants and be able to sit on the toilet and pee like everybody else. But now, when I need to go to the toilet, one of my friends pushes me there. Then she helps me on to the toilet and I hold on to her to balance and then she gives me the big bottle. My face is blushing as the yellow wee spills mostly into the bottle but some of it over my hand. I then worry whether the lost drops will affect my tests – and I wish the night was over.

Eventually I am driven home with the plastic container full of my urine sloshing in the back of the car.

The following morning I am allowed to miss church as I do not feel well at all. I feel sick and so, so tired. My head aches, for I did not sleep peacefully. The nightmares came to me again and again. Hellie is worried about my dreams and she tells Dad about them. He is angry with Dr Tan-Shoes. He storms around the house muttering under his breath and I feel guilty that maybe I have got the doctor into trouble. My sister stays at home and tells me my best friend, Adele, is coming to visit after lunch. I am looking forward to seeing her and I wait excitedly for her to arrive. She has written to me in hospital several times. Before I got sick, I was deputy head girl. Since my operation I have asked her to fill in for me.

She arrives looking as beautiful as ever, her long blonde hair curling neatly around her face. My mum and dad allow her to push me up to the park at the top of our road in the wheelchair. We sit in a derelict summer-house and chat together. My first question is about Martyn.

'How is my ex, then? Has he got a new girlfriend?'

'No. He's still cut up about what happened to you. I think he feels guilty.'

'Is he okay? I worry about him. He was special.'

'I know. Don't worry, I'm keeping an eye on him for you!'

'So what else has been happening? How did the mock A levels go?'

The exams for which I had studied so hard are now over, without me having a chance to take them.

Adele sighs heavily and dramatically. 'I failed physics spectacularly and so did Martyn. Vin-babes and John did really well and got A grades. Chemistry was all right – I passed that, and my biology too.'

She pushes me further along the winding path. I feel left out of the busy school routine and long to be back where I only have to worry about exams and homework.

'John has an offer at medical school,' she adds cautiously. 'He wanted to know if you had heard from any universities.'

'Yes, I have had offers from all of them now. I just have to choose my places, but I don't really know what to do – whether to go or not.'

'Why not?'

'Well, I don't even know if I'm going to make it, do I?'

'You should apply anyway. You have nothing to lose. You can always pull out. Anyway, you don't want John to get there first, do you?'

We laugh easily together. John and I always compete keenly for first place.

'But I will have missed so much work when I get back. I really don't know if I can take my exams. I feel so unsure of myself in every way these days and I feel scared whenever I think ahead. I begin to think maybe I'll tempt fate if I look into the future. I could make plans that will come to nothing.'

'Mary, you worked so hard for your mocks – you could pass your A levels tomorrow. Take them and see. You know the teachers will help you. We are all behind you, Mary, you know that.'

It is February now and more spring bulbs are breaking through. I think about the plan to save my tablets. As if reading my mind, Adele begins to speak again.

'You need to aim for something, Mary. You seem really down today. Next week it's Valentine's Day. How about aiming for that?'

'Yes, well, I know I won't be getting any cards.'

'Wait and see,' she says and smiles playfully. 'Maybe you'll get one from Barry.'

'No, I don't think so. I haven't written to him. I'll probably never see him again. There's no point.'

'You never know, maybe it's true love,' she says.

As she pushes me home, my life seems a little bit more normal – talking about exams and boys and Valentine cards. I amend my decision. I will save the tablets until I finish my chemotherapy and see how I feel then.

Okay, I tell my friend. I will aim for Easter.

'That's more like it,' she answers, and I find just a glimmer of hope.

I am full of trepidation as I make the journey back to Christie's on Monday. This time I know what terror awaits me. The nurses greet me cheerfully and ask me how the weekend went. I tell them about the brightly coloured berets and scarves and proudly show them off. I hand in my big container and await the results of my kidney tests. Dr Tan-Shoes comes to take my blood tests to check my bone marrow is not being damaged. I feel nervous waiting for the results. If my kidneys or my bone marrow fail then the chemotherapy will have to be delayed, which means the bad cancer cells could start to grow. I sit on my bed, biting my nails and worrying about the drugs. Shortly after breakfast, Vera approaches me.

'We've organized a surprise for you,' she says, seeing me unpack my nightdress. 'Don't put that on yet.'

'Where am I going?'

'To the artificial limb centre. We're going to get you a leg!' I look disbelievingly at her. I hadn't imagined this even in my wildest dreams! I had expected to be stuck in my chair or on my crutches for ages.

'A new leg! I can learn to walk again! I'll be able to see two feet again! I thought I would have to wait months for this!'

Vera joins in the general laughter. I am so elated and overwhelmed. Tears begin to flow, but this time they are tears of happiness.

'Well, last week we rang the doctor at the limb centre to check it out and he said to go straight along. Come on!'

She helps me into a waiting ambulance. Several other patients are already in the vehicle. None of them have two legs. All of them are old and look sick and disabled. An old man who is very overweight and out of breath looks curiously at me. I pretend to look out of the window. After a few minutes of awkward silence, he speaks to me.

'How did you lose yours, then?'

My heart races away. I have never met anyone else with a missing limb and I have never had to answer the question before. He doesn't seem bothered about his amputation but inside I feel again the agonizing stab of grief and loss. I so much want this to be a special day; I want to remember the day I first got my new leg – and yet it still hurts so much whenever I think of the leg that has gone. I pause, not knowing what to say and feeling angry he is treating the subject so casually.

'Mine was a blood clot,' he continues.

'Oh.' What else can I say?

What I want to say to him is this: 'Don't you understand what I have lost? Can't you feel my agonizing pain? Why are you blind to the mutilation of my healthy, beautiful body?'

'You're very young. Never seen anyone so young without a leg.' A smoker, he sucks in the air between a gap in his rotting teeth. He puffs and pants from the effort of too much talk and I can hear the rattle of his diseased lungs.

I hate him now, for I realize he had a choice and I had none. My leg was healthy and strong but the cancer came anyway. I look at him and despise him and his mistreated body.

The lady across from him is very thin with blue lips and doesn't have any legs at all. I look away in horror. How is it possible to be alive without any legs at all? I do not want to talk to old, sick people. I am young, too young for this. My anger rises.

Vera cuts in. 'Perhaps Mary doesn't want to talk about it. She has been very poorly.'

The man looks embarrassed and apologetic and I stare out of the window again with tears blurring the view. Soon we arrive at the limb centre and the ambulancemen help me to a smart waiting room. The old man and lady wheel over to a group of elderly people. They obviously know the routine. I feel disappointed. I thought I would meet some young people like me but everybody is old here too. I am relieved when I am called into the clinic to be introduced to a doctor and a man who explains he is called a prosthetist.

'My job is to make you an artificial leg,' he explains. 'The first one will be quite basic so you can learn to walk on it easily. Then, as you get better, we will update it.'

He leads me into a room full of bits of equipment. In the centre is a set of parallel bars at a low height.

'This is where you will learn to walk,' he continues. 'Our physiotherapist will help you.'

The doctor checks my Little Leg and leaves me with the prosthetist, who tells me to call him Mike.

'First thing we do is make a plaster cast,' he explains. 'Then we use that to make a little socket for your stump and we build the artificial leg around it.'

He takes a large bucket of water and soaks some messy plaster of Paris bandages which he wraps around my Little Leg, telling me to keep still until they set. Soon he shows me a perfect cast in the shape of my Little Leg.

'Right you are. Leave it with me and in two weeks we will have a leg for you.'

'Really? Is that it? What will it look like when it's done?'

He disappears to fetch one and returns with a leg under his arm. He plonks it unceremoniously on the floor. For the first time I see an artificial limb. It doesn't look too bad. It looks more or less like a leg. It is not a peg or anything terrible – just like a dummy leg in a shop window. He shows me how it works and hands it to me.

'Oh, it's so heavy!' My arms drop under its weight.

'That's the problem,' he explains sympathetically. 'You need to build up good strong muscles. This weighs much more than your own leg did, and now you have fewer muscles.'

'How long will it be before I can wear it?'

'Well, the plan is to wear it for a short time every day and build up your tolerance. The skin on your stump is not meant for walking on. It needs to toughen up. Maybe try an hour each day and then increase it. Within a few months you should be able to walk with the help of a stick.'

'But I thought it would take years to learn to walk!'

Mike laughs and I begin to feel hope returning.

'We'll have you up and about much sooner than that!'

On the way home I tell Vera enthusiastically about my morning.

'He was just so amazing! So clever and helpful. He is going to make me a leg and it will be ready in two weeks!'

It is well into the afternoon when I get back to Christie's. I am very tired. Vera tells me I need to rest on my bed. Inside myself I hide all the special things that have happened to me today at the artificial limb centre and yesterday at the park with Adele. I store up the good things like a squirrel preparing for winter days ahead. I will use the good things in the same way I use the antidote tablets to stop the chemo from killing me. If I think about good stuff then maybe bad stuff will not hurt as much.

By the evening I am bored and restless. I get up and wheel around in my chair. Then I spot my big brother, Martin, striding down the ward with a gang of friends.

'Hi there, Little Sis,' he says and whisks me off in the wheelchair down the corridor. His two friends, Vin and Adrian, each give me a bunch of red roses and a kiss on each cheek. The other ladies all tease me.

'We're taking you out – for Valentine's Day!' my brother explains.

'But you're not allowed!'

'Yes I am – I've okayed it with Sister Anna. Every Monday night I can take you out after your tests are complete!'

And so it becomes a weekly routine. Monday nights my brother and his friends take me off to have a little fun away from this strange dark world. They make me feel special and important but, most of all, they make me feel normal again.

The next day, when Dr Tan-Shoes arrives at my bedside with the needles and the drip bag, I close my eyes and remember the jollity and the jokes of the previous evening. I remember the romantic kiss that Vin playfully gave me. In fact, I replay the kiss many times during the next few days in between vomiting and retching. I recall the walk in the park with my best friend and imagine the new leg which is even now being built for me. I gaze at the vases of red roses and the cards that my physics class sent me for Valentine's Day. I put the one I received from Barry under my pillow and I dream about holding his hand in Ward Six. I think about the good things in my life and it helps. For this time the effects of the chemotherapy are worse. My body is poisoned a little more and I feel that much closer to death. It is as if I need to cling on to life and goodness. Only then can I overcome the effects of the poison.

At night, when I close my eyes and fall asleep, the bad stuff comes back and haunts my dreams. I see again the dogs and the gore of my leg being severed. Each morning I awake a little more exhausted and a little more desperate. When the yellow bag is finally taken away I truly wish that death would take me.

'Two lots of chemo down, four more to go,' says Dad on Thursday morning when he arrives to take me home. 'And it's your special weekend. All the family will be at home!'

I had never imagined my eighteenth birthday would be spent fighting cancer but I am determined to celebrate my special weekend in style. Who knows – it might be my last.

'Oh, and the doctors have decided to give you some new tablets to help your nightmares,' my dad tells me as he helps pack my case.

'What are they called?'

'Chlorpromazine. Only take them once you have got into bed at night. They are very, very strong.'

He gives me the box and I put them in my bag. In the car I try to decide what I will do with them. The nightmares are horrific … but I also need to save tablets. If I do decide to kill myself, I cannot run the risk of it going wrong. I decide I will break the tablets in half; that way I can help the nightmares and still have some to save.

When I get home I find my birthday weekend is to be packed with surprises. I have looked forward to becoming an adult for a long time but became one when they told me about my illness. I want to be a child again now. I have seen too much of the grown-up world and do not like it. My body should be turning into a woman's. But the chemotherapy has destroyed my ovaries and my womb. I am thin and my ribs stick out like they did when I was a little girl. My breasts have shrunk virtually to nothing. My periods have stopped and my body hair has fallen out completely. I guess soon my head will be bald, too. I am all smooth and pink and thin. It is scary, my body changing back to how it used to be before my periods started. So celebrating my eighteenth birthday feels quite strange. My mind feels as if it is sixty and my body feels about ten.

Friday, one by one, my brothers and sisters arrive home from school and college and university. They come and sit on my bed and tell me about the exciting times they are having. I wish that I had some normal, happy things to talk about. That night we three girls all push our beds together and I sleep safely in the middle and think maybe tonight the dogs won't attack me. But they do, even though I have taken half a tablet. I wake screaming, swearing and fighting and only stop when I realize it is Franny holding my fists.

'It's always like this,' I hear Hellie say. 'She's dreaming about dogs and that doctor she is so frightened of.'

My sister rocks me back and forth and I descend into a heavy, wretched sleep again.

Saturday dawns cold and bright and my sisters wake me gently. 'How about shopping for your birthday?' they ask me. I accept gratefully. Anything to take my mind off the black thoughts that overwhelm me after the nightmares. My instinct is to open the envelope I have carefully hidden in my box of private letters and swallow all the tablets, but I am worried that I do not yet have enough and my plan would fail. I'll have to wait. My sisters help me choose a beautiful dress for my birthday. Franny looks at me as she helps lift the soft cream taffeta over my shoulders.

'Mary, you're wasting away. There is nothing left of you.'

'I know,' I agree, 'but I just can't eat anything while I am having the drugs. Even when I get home I don't want to eat.'

71

'You look about six stone. And look at your ribs. I hate what they are doing to you.'

'I still have another four lots of chemo to go, as well. I feel so desperate inside. Like everything is black and hopeless.'

She kneels in front of me, her eyes filled with love. 'Don't give up, Mary. I know it's easy for me to say, but God is looking after you. I know He is going to get you through. Remember when you asked God to use you? Well, He will. Just hang on to that.'

I seem to have lost sight of God. I feel abandoned and betrayed by Him. When Franny and Irene talk about God, it's as if they are talking about a different God altogether. They talk about someone who is kind and loving. Yet when they try to explain, sometimes – just sometimes – I get a little glimpse of something that gives me hope. Just occasionally, I remember how the Presence felt. How I wish I could find my soul again but it has fled from me. All I feel is a terrible pit of despair. I fall into the foul stinking mess and cannot breathe. I want to claw my way back to the God I have lost, but I need a hand to pull me out. And there is no hand there. I am alone.

We go home with bags full of birthday shopping and I think how special I should feel, but I just feel ruined and tired.

Saturday night we all go out for a family meal.

'Mary, you're not eating much.' Franny cuts into my dark thoughts.

A wave of nausea sweeps over me and I stare unseeingly at the piece of birthday cake on my plate.

Now it is Sunday, and although my birthday is tomorrow, 20 February, we are celebrating today. Sunday is usually a rush first thing as we all prepare to go to Mass, but today my mum brings my breakfast on a tray. My sisters follow, carrying lots of cards and a huge pile of presents.

'Happy birthday to you!' they all sing. Outwardly I smile but inside my heart is breaking as I see my future so altered from what I had planned. How can I ever be happy again? My hopes lie shattered and I cannot even see as far ahead as next week, let alone another birthday.

I open my cards and gifts. There are so many that soon my sisters have to pile them up on their two beds as well. It makes it so hard, knowing I am loved so much, to contemplate ending my life. I read the kind words that friends and teachers – even strangers – have written, and feel ashamed that inside I am hiding so much. I feel so guilty that I want to die, but I just cannot help it. The thoughts appear in my head from nowhere.

'We've arranged a party for you today, Mary,' Hellie tells me excitedly. 'I can't keep it secret any longer. We've invited everyone from the God Squad and Adele has invited lots of your other schoolfriends.'

'And there is a secret surprise,' Franny tells me.

Hellie gets me ready, paying detailed attention to my hair and make-up. She stuffs padding down my bra. We giggle together as she stuffs some down her front, too. Franny and she have made an amazing cake for me – all pink and fluffy clouds. There is champagne, too! Soon the house fills with guests. My teachers turn up, including Mr Slack, who both Hellie and I have a massive crush on. He gives me some perfume and a card with a big kiss inside. The boys from my physics class arrive, John and Vin-babes. Even some of my brother's university friends make the trip from Manchester.

The party gets under way and my big brother fills up my glass with champagne and makes a speech. He says how proud he is of me and how courageous he thinks I am and tears fill my eyes. We have a wonderful time and Vin-babes and John make a big fuss of me. I feel normal and almost like a whole person again. Everybody is being very secretive about the surprise until at three o'clock the doorbell rings. Adele announces a surprise guest – and a huge furry gorilla enters the room, sits me on his knee and reads me a silly poem! We all laugh until the tears are rolling down our cheeks. I am presented with a red rose and a big kiss before he leaves.

After the buffet someone puts smoochy records on. A few girls get up and dance with the boys. I feel left out, rejected and ugly. I can't dance and, even if I could, nobody would want to dance with me. A sinking desperation sweeps over me and I hold back the tears.

Adele sits beside me. 'Don't worry,' she whispers. 'You will be dancing soon – when you get your new leg – and then there will be no stopping you!'

After the dancing finishes, John comes over to me. 'I wondered if I could take you for a push in your wheelchair?' he asks. He takes me out and shows me his new car. 'I passed my driving test,' he announces proudly, helping me in and loading the wheelchair before we set off for the park.

'What about medical school, then?' I ask him.

'I've chosen Birmingham first and Manchester second.'

'I've put down Sheffield and Liverpool.'

'You are going to take your exams, then? You must, you know. You worked so hard.'

'I don't know. I can't see that far ahead. I might not even …'

He glances at me quickly as my voice trails away.

'Yes, I know. But if you don't take them, you can't pass them.'

'What's the point, though, if I end up dying?'

'All the point in the world. It would be an achievement. Let's face it as well – the way our physics group is going you will be the only one to pass!'

We laugh together. I realize that being ill and talking to so many adults has made it a little bit easier to talk to boys. I could never have talked with John like this before.

'Adele and I will carve it on your gravestone,' he jokes, and suddenly it seems hilariously funny.

'Yeah, three As and a B at A level! Do you think we are really sick, making jokes like this together?'

'No … that's what med students do, isn't it? Honestly, Mary,' he says seriously, 'I'm not going to medical school without you. You have to fight this.'

'Okay, I'll try my hardest to fight.'

He pushes me round the park and I ask him to take me into the athletics stadium where I won the Victor Ludorum prize last sports day. John sits there in silence while I hunch up in the freezing cold with a blanket around my shoulders. I remember strolling around holding hands with Martyn in the blistering summer heat and how good it felt to push forward in the race with an easy stride and win.

John looks at me and smiles. 'You don't need to run to pass your exams,' he says.

On the way back to the car I set myself another goal. I had chosen Easter as a death date. Now I see it would be too early. I quite like the idea of taking my A levels, then killing myself and having something written on my gravestone. If I could last until then, I would have something to leave behind, something I could say I had done with my life.

'Okay,' I say to John in the car on the way home. 'I will take my exams. I mean, I probably won't pass them. But I promise I will take them.'

John and I say our farewells outside my home and shake on our deal.

'See you back in physics class.' He squeezes my hand.

Inside, they are waiting to say Mass. My friends have chosen all my favourite hymns and scriptures. I sing a chorus on my own and Mum starts to cry. Afterwards Martin and his friends prepare to return to university, but before they go they give me a big parcel.

74

'We've called him Henry,' they tell me as I unwrap an enormous cuddly hippopotamus. Henry is bright green with a yellow bow around his neck.

'He is for you to cuddle when you feel lonely in Christie's,' Martin tells me.

'We chose green so the sick wouldn't show up!' says Adrian, who is a med student and therefore allowed to make jokes like that.

It is awfully quiet as I sit in the lounge after the party. I tuck Henry under my chin and think about all that has happened today. I have a stay of execution again and my friend John has brought some hope into my colourless life. I decide to put some music on and, instead of calling someone, I do it myself. I stand up slowly and, balancing carefully on my one leg, I play my favourite Beatles record. I lean against the cool glass of the window pane and look outside, humming softly and listening to the words of 'Yesterday'. Later that night, before she leaves, Franny promises she will come and see me soon in hospital.

'I'll bring Pastor Tony, too. Remember now, be strong. We will get through it together. You, me and Hellie.'

She doesn't know how true her words are. We are all there together and I am drawing on the strength of my family and friends more than they will ever know.

6

Every week I have my chemo in Christie's and each time my body becomes a little more poisoned.

The third week of having treatment, I woke up one morning and sat up. There, on the pillow, lay clumps of my beautiful long hair. I screamed because I didn't know it would happen like that. Every time afterwards, when I brushed my hair, it fell out a bit more. I looked at my hairbrush and pulled out the thick strands which had been poisoned to death. My head was covered with bare patches which grew bigger and bigger each day until I looked like a balding sparrow.

Now, six weeks after starting chemo, I look like a baby bird, all bedraggled, with just fuzzy and sparse downy feathers.

And it wasn't just my hair that died. My eyebrows and my eyelashes died. My mouth and my eyes became poisoned and covered with dozens of tiny ulcers. My blood cells began to die, making me so weak that if I even caught a cold I could die and, from that point onwards, nobody has been allowed to come near me if they are sick. My veins have got worse every week and Dr Tan-Shoes gets more and more frustrated because he cannot find them. Last week it took him ten goes to get the drip in and I had to have some tablets afterwards to calm me down. My weight keeps falling and now I look like one of those children they show on *Blue Peter* when they are talking about famines and starving people. My body just throws the poison out all the time, whichever way it can. I vomit bright yellow, I wee bright yellow and I cry bright yellow.

Two weeks after my birthday I went back to the limb centre and picked up my new leg.

'Here we go,' Mike said. 'Let's try it on.'

I just put my Little Leg into the top of it. There are two belts to fasten it up. One big leather belt goes round my waist. That one is quite painful. Then another belt fastens over my shoulder and attaches to the waist belt.

'Okay, hold on to the bars and take a little step.'

'I can't. It's too heavy.'

'Come on, try. Use your back muscles, too.' So I tried my very hardest and I managed to move it. Then I took another step … and another. Mike showed me how to make the knee joint bend so I could sit down and how to lock it when I stand up.

'So now all you need do is take it away and practise. Wear it for half an hour more each day and the physiotherapist at Christie's will help you with your walking.'

I was surprised it was all so easy. I thought it would take years to learn to use an artificial limb.

So I took the leg back and dressed it up in my thick tights and shoe and put some fashionable leg warmers over the tights. You really couldn't tell it was an artificial limb – until I began to walk. When my brother visited in the evening with Vin and Adrian, I was sitting in my chair wearing my leg and waiting to surprise them! They were all so pleased they began to cry. Then they took me and Henry the hippopotamus out to celebrate. We always take Henry with us – he has become our mascot. Some of the nurses and doctors were out too and they came over and admired my leg. It is pretty difficult to put on. I need help because I can't balance and do up all the straps. But I have been practising very hard around the hospital and now I can wear it for quite a few hours at a time and walk a little way using my crutches.

But when I go home I get all the black thoughts and feelings that I want to die. I see this picture in my mind all the time when I am alone. I see snow, pure white and freshly fallen. Then I see a spreading stain of blood on the snow and feel relieved. I want it to be my blood. When I have the picture I get this urge to go and cut my body, maybe my wrist or maybe my throat. Then I could let my infected blood fall all over the snow. I looked at the kitchen knives the last weekend I was home but they are too blunt. I need a really sharp one. I can't do it, anyway, until after the exams. I made that promise to John and I want to keep it. I have saved lots of tablets now. I could take the tablets and then, before they work, let the blood out. That would definitely work. So that is what I think about a lot – death.

At the same time, there are so many things I want to do. Precious things like looking at daffodils in a park and drinking red wine from a crystal glass. Even while I am contemplating suicide, I also want to see life at all costs.

So, after two months at Christie's, my chemo is finishing right now. I am watching the last drops of yellow poison invade my veins. I am lying in my bed, counting the seconds until this last bag finishes. I am nearly dead but I have made it. I lie like a skeleton in a grave and think this is a living death. My sister visits me with Pastor Tony and I grip her hand and hold on to life. I talk to her about bad things but I cannot remember what I say. Her eyes darken as I talk to her. What am I saying? My brain is now poisoned, too. I try to draw some life from Franny. Even though I hate Dr Tan-Shoes, I could almost kiss him when he arrives to remove the chemo and pour the fresh clean salt water into my body so I can begin to become alive again.

At last I leave Christie's. My parents have a conversation with my doctor and they come out of her office with reddened eyes. But I do not care what has been said. It is over.

I am overjoyed to be home but there is a black and frozen emptiness inside my soul, like vast icy depths which threaten to drown me. Sometimes I can feel the pull downwards – death calling me. I try to fight the urge to close my eyes and surrender to its beckoning hand. Sometimes, when I get tired, a numb chilling fear enters my thoughts – perhaps I would be better off if I dipped my head beneath the surface for ever. But I promised, I promised not to give up. The Presence told me he would lead me through. Where is he? I need his hand again.

I hide away with the books that have become my friends. I have missed a lot of work. I need to catch up if I am to pass my exams. My teachers give me extra lessons. So I tuck myself away in a little study den I have created in Martin's room. Nobody is allowed in while I am studying, absolutely nobody. All my books and my notes are there. I sit for hours and hours, learning, reciting, revising for my big achievement. This is the prize which will be my epitaph. My parents let me study for endless hours. Mum brings me a steady supply of coffee. I do not go out at all. After studying, I lie on my big brother's bed with the curtains open. I can look out at the stars. I look out into the velvety darkness and my mind goes off wandering to strange and beautiful places. Sometimes to the past – running breathlessly around the park, skating crazily around the ice-rink and making long, tiring treks up mountains. Sometimes to where the future ought to be and what it would have been like to marry and be a doctor and have children. I am left wondering just how many good things have been denied me.

I hate going to Mass. I sit at the front of the church in my wheelchair. The words don't mean anything any longer, they are cold and harsh and empty. Anyway, my soul has died. Then I start to cry. I always cry. It feels like I am crying blood and sometimes I wish I was: chalices of my bad and evil blood poured out over the clean, white altar cloth.

Easter is approaching. Afterwards I shall go back to school. I have worked and worked in my den. I have found solace in atoms and molecules, in formulae and symbols. I am holding on for the final day of my exams.

Every week I return to Christie's for my check-up. They take X-ray pictures of my chest to look for secondaries. Each time I go there I feel so frightened at what they might find. So far it's okay. The cancer has not grown back. It is not going to kill me yet.

Just before Easter, I receive an appointment to visit the Artificial Limb Centre at the Royal Preston Hospital. I don't want to go. There seems no point. I will not need to walk after the exams. I will be gone from here. I cannot tell my parents that so, when they arrange for me to visit, I have to make the trip.

When I arrive, it is just like the time I went to Manchester. The centre is full of old, sick people in wheelchairs. I look around and feel dull black inside. I should not be here. The old people chat and discuss their operations. I sit dozing in my wheelchair and ignore them, pretending to be asleep when the conversation turns towards me.

'Hey, wake up, sleepy-head!' I open my eyes to see a short man with an enormous beard. His face is tanned and the lines around his eyes give away how much he laughs. His hands are large and covered in cuts and plasters. 'Don't fall asleep – we've got work to do!'

He takes my wheelchair and pushes me quickly up the corridor into a fitting room. It looks familiar – bars down the middle, large mirror at each end of the bars and a couple of chairs. An assortment of false legs lies cluttered around. My heart sinks again.

'Right. I'm your prosthetist from now on. I used to mend cars and now I mend legs!' It is hard not to smile. 'We are going to get to know each other quite well, so you call me John and I'll call you Mary. Okay with you?'

'Sure.'

79

'So you had a bone tumour – which meant surgery and chemotherapy, yes? Well, we're not here to talk about cancer. I'm sure you've had enough of that. What about you? What do you want to do?'

'I've got a place to do medicine. I want to be a doctor – if I make it.'

'Kid, you will if you fight for it. But didn't it put you off, all the treatment?'

'No. It has made me see what makes a good doctor.'

'That's my girl, good for you,' he says. 'So we need to get you up and about for the start of the new university year.'

'Do you think I can do it, then? Be a doctor?'

'Mary, I have this saying. Never say you can't do something until you've given it a bloody good try. So how are you feeling about your leg?'

'I feel horrible most of the time. Not so much about losing my leg – more the cancer and not being able to do what I used to.' I quickly brush the tears away from my eyes.

'Look,' he says gruffly. 'I'm not very good at this bit, but look at what you could achieve if you fight for it. You've got the chance to become a doctor. Make it your goal. Have you ever been good at sport?'

'Yes, I was really good. It's one of the things I miss – running and gym, things like that.'

'Well, look at it as if it were a race. Practise, train and keep your eyes on the finishing post. I can make you the best leg around but you have to want to get up and walk. Think you can do it?'

'Yes. I think I can.'

'Right. Now I don't think you're walking very well. And your belt sticks out a mile. Makes you look all lopsided. We can't have that.'

'I didn't think it mattered what my leg looked like. Isn't it more important to be able to walk?'

'Of course it matters how you look. When you buy a pair of shoes you don't buy them just for comfort, do you? You need them to look good, too. Well, it's the same with legs. I make them look good and walk good.'

He helps me remove my artificial leg and leaves the room with it draped over his shoulder, whistling as he goes.

He returns with some plaster of Paris bandages and a couple of big buckets of water. Then he disappears again and returns with a huge piece of paper and assorted rulers.

'I'm starting again,' he says as he soaks the bandages. 'That leg isn't right for you. I can do you a better one.' He whistles all the time and as he shapes the creamy plaster he considers his work proudly.

'It's a craft, this,' he confides. 'You have to love it.' His calloused hands smooth the cast into shape and, by the time he has completed his sculpture, I feel proud, too.

'Okay, now lie down on the paper,' he says, and I giggle.

'Seriously?'

'Yes. I'm going to draw around your right leg so we can match it up to your prosthesis. We can't have you with huge muscles on one side and nothing on the other.'

He helps me sit on the paper and draws a tracing of my leg.

'That's it. Come back in two weeks and your leg will be ready for you. Meanwhile, I've done a beauty job on your old one!' He leaves the room and waves farewell to me, walking away with a spring in his step.

It is the week before Easter and I am impatient for it to be over. I have two things to aim for – getting my leg from John and going back to school. First, though, I have to get Easter out of the way. The endless gloomy services loom in my thoughts. It also means I have to go to confession. I am getting more and more confused about the suicide plan. I decide to confess to saving up the tablets. I know it is wrong to take them. Perhaps, with it being Easter, if I confess about the tablets then I will find God again and my soul will begin to live once more. So, on Palm Sunday, when Dad takes us to the usual pre-Easter confessions, I take the big brown envelope, now full to bursting, and put it in my bag.

I confess to contemplating a mortal sin – taking my own life – and hand over the tablets to a priest. I utter the prayer I learnt when I was seven years old about being sorry and trying not to sin again. I say a penance and am forgiven.

Good Friday dawns with the sunshine streaming through the windows. It is a day for being serious and quiet. Usually we have to fast but this year I am excused because of being so ill. It doesn't really make a difference. I fast every day now.

Hellie helps get me ready for church. We sit on the bed together and she combs the sparse remains of my hair. The strands are still coming out and they fall on to my dress. I am impatient for my new hair to start growing again. I hate looking so bizarre.

'Pick the hair off my dress, Hellie. It's driving me wild.' She starts to brush the hair off and soon there is a large pile. She fixes some pretty slides she has made to hide the worst patches but, as she does so, more hair falls out.

'I hate this, I really do. It is so horrible. When will it grow again?'

'I don't know, Mary, I'm sorry.' She begins to remove the hair from my dress again and I pick up the hairbrush and throw it across the room. It hits the wall with a loud thud. Hellie walks over patiently and picks it up without saying a word. When she comes back, I see she is crying, too.

'I just want you to be better, Mary,' she weeps. I realize she is tired and worried. Every night I wake her with my screams and punches. I feel guilty again for causing her so much pain.

The Good Friday service is cold and gloomy. The flowers are all taken away from the altars and the statue of Christ is covered with a black cloth. The story of the Passion of Christ is read and parishioners read out the spoken parts: Barabbas, Pilate and Judas Iscariot. Then we all go up to the altar. I hate this bit. We kneel in front of it and have to kiss the feet of the metal figure of Jesus nailed to the wooden cross. When I get to the crucifix I am shaking. Suddenly I break down. I start to cry and shake as Dad hastily escorts me out into the priest's house. I am screaming and shouting, 'Why, God? Why?' at the top of my voice. I am crying hysterically about my leg and the cancer and my beautiful hair. I am crying about babies and chemotherapy and all that was so special.

Dad settles me on a sofa and brings me a cup of hot, sweet tea. One of the ladies of the parish comes in and offers to sit with me while my dad returns to the service. The lady is kind and she prays as I lie exhausted on the sofa. I hear the final chords of the closing hymn drift through from the church and tidy my dishevelled appearance. I sink once more into a pit of dark, black despair.

Easter Sunday morning is bright and fresh. I wonder perhaps whether the new life promised by this holy day will bring new hope for me too. As I prepare for church I think about how I felt on Friday and then I remember that in the Bible the dark gloom of Good Friday became the joy of the first Easter Sunday. I also recall that the last big feast at church was Christmas Day and I think how much has happened since then. I was filled with happiness and my life had new meaning and seemed so perfect. Now it is changed beyond recognition. Everything is different – my body, my life, my faith.

The Easter holidays drift by and soon it is time to return to school. I now have my second artificial limb – and John is right, it is much better. It fits more closely and I do not look all lumpy. It is not quite so heavy and I can manage to walk short distances if I use both my crutches. It is also much more comfortable to wear. John Jackett has done as he promised – he has built me the best leg he can. If I dress it up with thick grey tights, it looks pretty realistic.

I feel excited at the prospect of returning to my studies but it is nerve-racking to think of meeting my friends again. The last time I was at school, I walked along the corridors on two strong, healthy legs and ran out on to the hockey pitch at lunchtime. Now I can only hobble painfully and slowly with my artificial leg. Our school is very old and draughty, with long stone staircases, and I am worried about getting around. I will have so many explanations to give and, in physics, I will have to see Martyn again.

It is a very strange feeling when I put on my sixth-form uniform for the first time this year. It is almost five whole months since I last wore it. I could not have imagined what lay ahead of me when I hung up my smart grey skirt for the Christmas holidays and took the deputy head girl's badge off my black jumper. Now, as I contemplate the future and my exams, I feel as if the very foundations of my world have been shaken. My dad drives me to school and leaves me with the secretaries. They all crowd round me and welcome me back. The headmaster, Mr McCarthy, arrives and chats with me about the term ahead.

'Just do what you are able,' he tells me. 'If you are too tired to go to a lesson then either go home or work quietly in the library.'

Adele joins me shortly afterwards, ready to escort me to my first lesson – biology. As we walk through the doors I am overwhelmed by the familiar sharp smell of formaldehyde. It is pungent but very different to the antiseptic smell of the hospitals I have lived in for the last few months.

'It's rat dissection at the moment,' Adele explains.

The biology lab is exactly as I left it; the same posters line the walls, the blackboard is still half-dusted and Mr Johns' white lab coat hangs on the same old hook. It reminds me of Dr Jimmy in his white coat, laughing and joking, and I remember his encouragement to study hard. Adele and I take up our usual table and put the jotter in between us in case we need to write each other notes.

'Are you okay?' she asks.

'I'm doing fine,' I say. And I am. It is wonderful to be back, although I feel a little apprehensive at the thought of how much work I have missed. Mr Johns comes over and welcomes me back to the class, promising me help if I need it. My class-mates arrive and some of them come over and greet me. John and Vin-babes wave.

Our first lesson is to carry on with the rat dissection. Adele has already started. Mr Johns hands out the sharp knives, and as he gives us ours I feel a stab of fear.

'Do you want to cut?' asks Adele. 'You need to practise for medical school.'

'No, you start,' I say, and swallow hard as she wields the knife. The thought of a blade cutting through skin and flesh is too difficult.

The next lesson is double physics and I have new hurdles to face. I have to see Martyn again. Adele knows I feel worried. I also feel embarrassed because I look so strange with my old hair almost completely gone and my downy new hair still growing back.

'Do I look all right?' I whisper to her.

'You look beautiful,' she says. 'You look calm, serene and composed – truly wonderful!' I feel so grateful to my friend.

'He's arrived,' whispers Adele and puts the notebook in between us. 'How do you feel?' she writes.

'Nervous!' I scrawl.

'Ignore for a while,' she jots. 'Then flash big flirty smile!'

When I feel brave enough, I turn my head and look at him. I smile shyly and lower my eyes briefly. He smiles back, but there is sadness in his eyes. I wish I could take away his guilt.

The lesson progresses and I see I have a lot of work to catch up on. My head is spinning by the end of the lesson and I am exhausted by the end of the day. I also make it to chemistry, sedately carried up two flights of stairs to the lab by Mr Slack and Mr McCarthy.

'This is just a ploy, isn't it – to get Mr Slack to sweep you off your feet!' Adele jokes. We laugh together and I feel so happy to be back at school. I enjoy the practical. I sit on the stool giving Adele directions while she attempts to blow up the science lab with ether! It seems like the first fun I have had in a long time.

Back home, after supper and a rest, I head up to my den to study.

'Don't overdo it, Mary,' my mum says gently. 'Remember, it is your first day back.'

'I won't, Mum, but I really need to catch up on my physics. I'll be working late.'

And so the pattern is set. I work hard at my lessons in school and continue at home in my den. I blot out the awful memories with chemistry equations and physics formulae. My biology file fills up with reams of meticulously illustrated notes. Soon I have finished all the practice exam papers and my teachers have to set more questions for me. I cocoon myself in a private unreachable world.

At school I do not join in much with the God Squad stuff any more. When they meet at lunchtimes I go to the library and say I have to work. Soon my marks are the highest in the year again. In May I begin the serious final sprint towards my exams. I study from dawn until late at night. My parents worry about the amount of time I spend in my den but I love the escape into my books. They are so safe and pre-dictable. The days roll into each other as I read my notes and textbooks from cover to cover. I continue to work alone, reciting my physics formulae over and over again as if in a dream.

The death thoughts have diminished since I returned to school, although I still feel black and empty when I am alone and not busy. I am still expecting to die from cancer. I still get so scared of it coming back. I check every night as I lie in my bath, prodding my limbs and tummy for lumps. When I wake up I rub my hands over my skin to see if I can find any Limpets. Every week I hold my breath as I return to Christie's for a check-up, but my doctors are pleased so far. I don't pray any more, only when I have to, at Mass. I don't really think God wants me now. There must be something wrong with my soul that makes bad things happen. So I say the right words when people ask me but, really, I have lost faith. It feels as if Jesus has turned His back on me. My thoughts, my mind, have grown dull and heavy. It is as if someone has taken a paint-brush and painted everything I think and know and feel in black. This is a tunnel of gloom and misery through which I trudge mechanically. The end of the journey is after the exams; then I am going. I collect my achievement for the gravestone, then I take my life. I have no life left, anyway. Once I have finished with my learning then what do I have left? No body, no future, no God.

I take an overdose one bleak day when things seem particularly ter-rible. It is a half-hearted attempt. All I can find is a handful of sleeping tablets. On the spur of the moment and desperate to escape my black thoughts, I swallow them, wishing I had more. My dad notices my slurred speech and I admit what I have done. My parents are not angry, as I thought they would be. They tuck me up in bed and one of dad's doctor friends comes to check my breathing and blood pressure. I sleep for a long, long time – a deep, dreamless sleep. The following day I am taken to see another doctor. I am led into a dark, shady room with a couple of big leather couches. There are strange, dark pictures on the wall. I talk to a middle-aged man who wears a suit, not a white coat. He tells me he is a psychiatrist. He is very kind and understanding. He thinks I am depressed and so he gives me some anti-depressants. My dad checks the packet every day.

One day, while I am locked away in the den, my dad comes to talk to me.

'Mary,' he says, 'one of your friends has been asking for you.'

'Oh?'

'It's Peter … from Ward Six. He is very ill. His head injury has not really improved and he is in another hospital. He was asking for you to visit.'

'I'm busy.'

'He was never too busy for you, was he?'

I know my dad is trying to get me to leave my den but I do not want to go outside.

'Shall I take you down to see him?'

I owe the boys from Ward Six. They helped me.

'Okay.' I get up to go and make myself look a bit more presentable, and soon we are heading towards South Shore Hospital, which is a rehabilitation unit. Dad shows me where to go and then promises to collect me in an hour. I knock softly on the door of Peter's room.

'Come in!' calls a cheery voice and shyly I peer round the door.

'Mary! Come and have some vodka!' I laugh – it seems like the first time in weeks – as I remember the celebration with my friends.

'It's so good to see you,' says Peter. 'We all missed you so much after you left hospital. When we didn't hear from you, we wondered if you'd made it. Then my mum bumped into your dad and he said you were back.'

'Yes I'm back, but my hair isn't!'

'It looks punky,' he jokes. Soon I am laughing again at his constant teasing. We talk together for ages and he shows me his paintings. He is an artist and his room is piled high with paper, paints and half-finished works. After I have admired them, he looks at me with a mischievous grin.

'There's someone else here who would like to see you.'

'Who might that be, then?'

'Barry.' I stare at him, lost for words. Peter adds, 'He's next door!'

'Barry is next door and you've only just told me? I can't believe it!'

'See you later, Mary,' he teases and waves goodbye. I knock on the neighbouring door, my heart pounding excitedly. I hear Barry's voice and my spirits soar.

'I knew you were here!' he said. 'I haven't heard Peter laugh like that for ages!' He holds his arms out to me and I walk over and sit on his bed. 'You look so lovely,' he says to me, and I lie with my cheek on his chest as he smoothes my short new hair.

'I missed you,' he whispers to me.

'I missed you, too,' I say, and stay there, quietly listening to the beat of his heart, until it is time to leave. He kisses my head softly and I feel safe again. There is no need to talk. We have both been through our different traumas and now we have found each other again. We do not need to explain.

'I'll see you tomorrow,' I promise.

So my life takes another turn and the blackness begins to lift. Barry has broken his leg again and will be in hospital for a long time. I visit him daily after I have finished my studies. I spend the evenings with him and he spurs me on. As the exams approach he fills me with courage.

'You can do it, babe,' he tells me and kisses me for good luck. 'You'll be a doctor one day, I know it.' We talk and talk until we know a lot about each other. We laugh and hug and kiss. We are in love. And with love, the dark clouds scatter.

My exams start and I make a little calendar for myself. I am looking forward to the day when I can cross out the last exam and spend uninterrupted time with Barry. One by one I score through the subjects with bold red felt pen. My hard work seems to have paid off and I find biology and chemistry easier than expected. I mess up the physics paper a bit, but I think I do well enough to make my grade.

I walk out into the sunshine after my last exam with an overwhelming sense of relief. Finished at last! I think maybe I have done quite well and now I need to decide about the future. Today was the day I had planned to end it all – I thought of stealing sleeping tablets from the medicine cupboard at home, walking down to the promenade, taking the tablets and jumping into the sea. Then Barry came back into my life and now we have such fun together. He makes me feel loved and special. He doesn't notice my leg and he thinks my hair looks cute now it is growing back all curly and soft. When he kisses me it takes away some of the bad memories and I feel cleaner than I did. So as I walk away from my last exam with my friend Adele, she asks me what I will do to mark the occasion.

'I think I will go and visit Barry,' I tell her. 'I'll smuggle something in for us to celebrate!'

I postpone my plans to go to the promenade. I will just wait for my results, I decide. Maybe by then I will have some idea of what the future holds.

But despite my happiness with Barry, the black thoughts keep returning. I begin to write poems. They are my suicide notes. Nobody knows how I feel inside. I starve my body. Sometimes I am happy. When I am with Barry I am happy. Life is so simple with him. It is like love should be. Clean, easy and honest. But I also have moments when I can see no way through and so I leave the poems lying around. Maybe someone will realize how I feel. To me they seem so obvious. I write about dying. I draw pictures of me with no leg and no womb and my head split in two, which is how I feel. I cry out for help, but it is as if nobody is listening. They are waiting for something else. They are waiting to hear the sound of the army of bad cells advancing again. Thoughts and minds are turned to the Limpet. Yet this is my real death.

One Sunday I go to an evening service in Fleetwood. I sit a couple of rows from the front and stare at the statues of the Virgin. Towards the end of the Mass I feel a strange emptiness in my head. The world goes black and very, very silent. When I come to, I am on the floor. My limbs ache all over. I feel bruised. I try to focus but I am unable to see straight. I see lots of tiny spots in front of my eyes. I am whisked off to Christie's the following day for a check-up. My dad talks in lowered tones to a doctor. He thinks I can't hear, but I can. The doctor thinks I don't understand, but I do. I hear the doctor talking about my brain. I hear him talk about my prognosis. I hear him talk about secondaries and he uses the word 'hopeless'. This is it, then. My brain is full of the Limpet's offspring. I am dying.

I don't care. Dying is better than living. I just don't care.

To ward off the black thoughts, I plough all my energies into visiting Barry.

'It's the school summer leavers' ball next week,' I tell him. 'Do you think you'll be out of hospital?'

'No, I don't reckon I will be.'

I look disappointed, so Barry tries to cheer me up. 'Tell you what. You come here before the ball. Put your dress on and come and show me what you look like. Maybe I'll get some champagne smuggled in as well!'

The days fly by and soon Friday arrives. It is a beautiful July day, hot and sunny. I spend hours doing my hair which has grown back quite well. Hellie does my make-up and I put on a gorgeous dress Adele has designed and made for me. It is golden honeysuckle yellow with layers and layers of soft silk petticoats and tiny pearly buttons. My mum lends me some jewellery. Then I am ready and I go to the hospital to see Barry.

'Have a wonderful night, babe,' he says. I wave and blow him a kiss.

'See you tomorrow!' I call.

Everybody is at the ball – our teachers, the secretaries and all our year. After the meal we get up to dance. I can't dance properly but I have been practising with Adele. John asks for the first dance and I accept. We sway to the music and have such fun. After that I am not short of partners and my dress is admired by everybody. I even have a dance with Mr Slack! The night flies by and I am dizzy with dancing and gin and tonic by the time the last number comes around. I wonder nervously if I will have to sit this one out. There is a tap on my shoulder and I turn to see Martyn.

'For old times' sake?' he asks. I put my head on his shoulder as he pulls me close and whispers in my ear.

'I'm so sorry,' he says. 'I'm sorry I hurt you and sorry about what happened to you.'

'It's okay. It's not your fault. It was just lousy timing.'

I feel him relax in my arms and know I have just eased his burden of guilt. We hug and everything is mended.

It is a strange feeling when the dance ends. We all say our goodbyes and go our separate ways. My schooldays are over now. It should be a time to look to the future and yet the future seems so uncertain. I never anticipated I would leave school with the dark shadow of death looming over me.

Later, back home, as I undress in my little den, I sit on the small bed and look out into the darkness. This room has been my refuge during so many hours. I have looked out of the window and my mind has travelled to all sorts of different places in an attempt to escape the horror. At this moment I decide I shall conquer and not surrender. I am eighteen. I am too young to give in. Too much lies ahead. It is time to leave this place of despair and never return ...

The hot summer begins. There is much work to be done. I need to learn to walk again. My rehabilitation has suffered while I have been revising. Now I need to become mobile – and quickly! If I pass my exams and go to medical school I will need to be able to walk between lectures. My sisters promise to help. Franny is home from physiotherapy college and Hellie has also finished her exams. My parents take us away for a holiday in the Cotswolds. We have rented a beautiful old gatehouse cottage on a large country estate. We three girls share a room just as we do at home. The sun beats down every day and Hellie and Franny encourage me to do more and more. Using a single crutch, I practise hard to build up my stamina and strength. Together we walk around the overgrown gardens, negotiating steps and rough ground. Franny issues me with instructions.

'You need to stand straighter, Mary.'

'I'm trying my best.'

'Come on, try harder. You look all lopsided!'

Each day we walk a little further and I manage to wear my leg a bit longer. Sometimes I abandon my crutches, link arms with my sisters and feel a little less self-conscious. One day on our walk we discover a large stone building. Inside there is a deep, inviting swimming pool.

I have always been an excellent swimmer but since my operation I have found it so hard to swim. I have been to a pool twice but could not bear the cringing, awkward embarrassment of entering the pool on my crutches, with my amputation so obvious to all. And then the left side of my body was so weak I could not go straight. I became upset and wanted to cry.

Franny mentions the pool to my dad who later comes back with the good news that we can use it as much as we like. We march off together to try it out.

'Okay, Mary,' says Hellie briskly. 'You're first in!' They help me remove my artificial leg and I slide into the pool, feeling the freedom of floating in water. Tentatively, I take a few strokes but I still veer off to one side. I always swim breaststroke and it is difficult with only one leg, although it is lovely to move again without the weight of my false leg.

My dad watches from the side of the pool. 'Try front crawl,' he suggests. 'Your arms are so much stronger now.'

So I try … and feel my arms cutting through the water, propelling my body in a straight line. 'It works!' I yell back. 'Come and teach me front crawl!'

Soon I am ploughing up and down the pool effortlessly. As my confidence grows again, I learn to duck and dive. Soon I am as good a swimmer as I have ever been.

I become braver. I draw strength from my sisters and we live out the pact to share our legs. Towards the end of the holiday we visit a beautiful gorge with waterfalls to admire. The rocks are slippery and gleaming with spray. My parents watch warily from the top while Hellie, Franny and I make our way down. I use my crutches and Hellie walks in front to clear the path. Franny grabs hold of the back of my trousers in case I should fall. At a painstakingly slow pace we make cautious progress and eventually turn a corner to see a beautiful waterfall cascading over a cliff edge. A rainbow catches the sun.

'Worth it?' Hellie asks.

'Yes, oh yes!' I reply, exhausted but happy.

Several hours later we arrive back at the top to meet our parents. 'I made it!' I say breathlessly and filled with pride. My parents laugh together, relieved to see us in one piece.

'It's hard to let you go and do these things,' my dad confides later. 'But we are truly very proud of you!'

That night, my sisters and I sit out together under the stars. Franny has brought her guitar and we sing together. Hellie and I lie on our backs, looking up to the sky.

'Do you remember last year?' I ask them. 'When we sat and sang by the lake?' They both recall the moment.

'The night seemed perfect,' says Hellie. 'Do you remember how we all ran down the mountain holding hands?'

'Yes, I miss that so much – running together. We won't do that again.'

'Who says?' challenges Franny.

'I can't run any more.'

'Not on your own.'

'Do you think Mary could run if we helped her, then?' Hellie questions.

'We can only try.'

'What if I fall?'

'We won't let you.'

'I agree,' says Hellie. 'We can support you.'

'You reckon it would work?'

'Definitely. Let's give it a go!'

So we link arms, they run and I try with all my might. Soon we are flying through the air! I am half skipping, half jumping and half being dragged along – but it feels like running. Breathlessly we collapse in a pile, laughing.

'I don't know what I would do without you!' I giggle.

Soon after our return from holiday, I am packing my suitcase again. My destination this time is Lourdes in France. I am going on a pilgrimage to the shrine of Our Lady, where miracles happen and there is a stream to bathe in. The water is said to be holy and supposedly has healing powers. I know now that my leg will not grow back, but maybe I could pray that my cancer will be cured. On arrival, I see a very tall young man pushing through the crowd towards me.

'Hi, Mary!' he greets me. 'I'm Jean-Paul, just done first year med at Cambridge. I hear you're hoping to be a med student too. I've been allocated to show you round the sights.'

The first evening he takes me to the grotto of Our Lady where St Theresa is said to have seen the vision of the Blessed Virgin. It is approaching midnight when we arrive at the small cleft in the rock where a statue marks the site. There are dozens of pairs of crutches hanging from the rock. Jean-Paul points to them: 'You can leave yours here next year!' he jokes.

'Now I'm taking you to see something really special!' he says, and we head away from the grotto towards a wooded path. I hear the distant sound of music and smell bonfires. Through the trees I glimpse bright colours whirling around and, as I get closer, I see there are dancers. They are beautiful with olive skin and long dark hair. They twirl around, wearing ornate dresses and playing tambourines.

'Who are they?' I ask Jean-Paul.

'Romany Christians. They are here on pilgrimage, too.'

We settle down on the edge of the gathering and some of the Romany people beckon to us to come closer. Jean-Paul pushes my wheelchair nearer to the bonfire. The Romanies are singing hymns and dancing, wearing garlands of flowers, and they seem so full of joy. Suddenly a silence settles and they begin to pray in French. I feel a sense of peace settle over me and my parched soul drinks in the silence. A young man stands up to share his story and Jean-Paul translates for me.

'He is telling us how Jesus came into his life and transformed him from an old to a new life,' he says, whispering the translation, and something inside me rekindles and grows.

When the young man has finished we wave goodbye to our friends and Jean-Paul pushes me back towards the hotel. But we have only gone a short way when we hear someone running after us.

'Excusez-moi, mademoiselle, monsieur!'

Jean-Paul stops and speaks with the young man who told his story. 'He has a prophecy for you, Mary,' Jean-Paul explains.

The young man leans down until he is level with my chair and speaks quietly to me in broken English. He looks into my eyes intently and, as he speaks, I become aware of my heart beating rapidly.

'You be okay – Jesus, He heal you. You have some children one day.'

I shake my head. 'No, I can't have any. The doctors told me.'

The young man looks at me, smiling broadly, his teeth flashing white in the darkness. 'Jesus – He can do anything, yes? You have a boy and a girl. Believe, yes?'

I smile at him and he runs back silently into the wood. The night has been so special and I tuck the memories away inside my heart, hoping and praying with all my life they are true.

On the day of departure I say tearful farewells to all my new friends, especially Jean-Paul. I have grown in courage and found a new belief in myself at Lourdes. That in itself feels like a miracle after the months of fighting fear. The feelings of deep despair are fading into the past and I am looking forward to going home.

The day of the A level results dawns and I wake early. Martin greets me and offers to take me to school. I have accepted a place at Liverpool University and need two B grades and a C. We head down to the sixth-form building. My brother chats away cheerfully, trying to distract me. Groups of students are already gathered as we arrive and join the queue. John is waiting in front of me. He has a place at Birmingham and needs three Bs. I remember the promise I made him – to sit my exams – and also recall the suicide I contemplated. A shiver goes through me as I fleetingly revisit those dark days. My brother sees it.

'Are you feeling okay?'

'Just nervous.'

'You'll be fine, I know. If anyone deserves to pass, it's you.'

As John's turn arrives to collect his results he smiles at me. 'Wish me luck!'

'Good luck, then, but I know you've passed!'

I wait anxiously for my friend. Several minutes later he comes out, joyfully waving his slip of paper.

Now it's my turn and I walk slowly forward on my crutches. Soon I will know what is in store for me. I push open the door of the headmaster's study and make my way inside, my heart beating nervously. I have battled for this moment and, as it arrives, my life moves in slow motion.

Mr McCarthy is saying something but I cannot make out what it is and I sit down heavily in the chair. He is handing me a slip of paper and I take it mechanically, my mouth dry and my palms sweating. This is the moment for which I have studied all my school life. I cannot focus on the writing and, as I try to take in what my headmaster is saying, tears spring to my eyes and the results blur.

He speaks again: 'Considering what you've been through ...'

I stare down at the slip of paper. My tears fall and soak it as my future unfolds ...

7

'You must be Mary from Blackpool!'

I turn and look up at a fellow student. He grins and thrusts out his hand. Awkwardly I remove mine from my crutches and feel his warm, confident handshake. He seems totally unconcerned by the newness of our surroundings. I am feeling completely out of my depth. The entire freshers' year of Liverpool Medical School has been herded into a small room in the pre-clinical building for our first anatomy practical. Wednesday morning anatomy practicals will be part of my routine for the next two years – if I make it. The sword always hangs over me; I never forget it. I have just learned to push the thought to the back of my mind.

The two days since I arrived have been a round of meeting other students, buying bits and pieces for my bright new room in Dale Hall and attending various rowdy freshers' parties. Today is the day I have been waiting for all summer since I heard the great news about my A level results. For today is the day that medical school starts for real and lectures begin.

A warm feeling rushes over me as I recall the interview with my headmaster, Mr McCarthy, back in August. I just exploded with pride when I saw I had three A grades, with a C in physics, and had passed my special papers in chemistry and biology. John had waited outside for me and as soon as I saw him we gave each other a hug. That was the moment I started to live fully again after the dark days I had been through.

Now I feel incredibly nervous and overawed by the large number of med students milling around. I am very conscious of my crutches, my bulky limb and my crop of baby, tightly curled hair, now growing back. Gratefully, I turn to make conversation.

'Yes, I am Mary from Blackpool – but how do you know that?'

'My mum is a nurse at Christie's. She told me to look out for you. Apparently you're quite famous there!'

'Well …' I hesitate, not wishing to reveal the terror I still feel when I hear the name of the hospital.

'My mum told me about this amazing girl who fought bone cancer, lost a leg and still managed to pass her A levels with flying colours in the space of a year. Could that be you?' He smiles cheekily, his head on one side, regarding me quizzically. I laugh and give in.

'Okay, it sounds like me.'

'I'm John Kirwan, from Manchester. Or Big John to my friends. It's a pleasure to meet you. I want you to know that if you need anything, just give me a call. I'm under strict instructions from my mum!'

'I will, Big John!'

'So tell me this incredible story, how you managed to pass your A levels after all that.'

So I tell him about the bone cancer and the amputation, the chemotherapy making my hair fall out and my new artificial leg. We joke together about it. It is wonderful just to be accepted as I am. I am no longer 'tragic Mary'. I'm just 'Mary from Blackpool'. It feels great.

A couple of other students approach. Big John is obviously well known already. He introduces me to a crowd, explaining quite naturally why I am using crutches, and they look at me curiously. One of the girls greets me enthusiastically.

'It's great to meet you,' she says. 'I'm Alison. We're dissection partners – I've just seen the notice board. I hope you're brainy! Have you seen the book we need to use? It's completely awful!'

Dissection is the first hurdle med students have to face. Four work together at one table which gets allocated a dead body, or cadaver, and over two years the cadaver is totally dissected. That is how we learn the anatomy of the human body. The older students have been regaling us with dissection stories. I think most of us are feeling very apprehensive. The smell of formalin is overpowering in the stuffy room and it reminds me of the hospital smells with which I have become so familiar. The second years told us this story about one girl who went into the anatomy lab only to discover that her cadaver was her grandmother! We were all totally horrified and I told my dad about it on the phone last night. He laughed and said: 'That story is told to every new med student year! It's all part of the tradition.'

'Are you squeamish, Mary?' asks Alison. 'I'm worried in case I faint.

Some of the second years told me that every year someone faints. I hope it isn't me.'

'No, I'm not squeamish,' I say. But I do remember the sound of the old lady dying. I have heard death but never seen it. Now I will see it.

Suddenly the lab doors open and two middle-aged ladies come in.

'I'm Joan,' the first lady says in a broad Scouse accent.

'And I'm Rita,' adds the other lady in even broader Scouse.

'We're the dissection technicians. Any problems, come and find us. Make a queue and we'll give you each a white coat and a dissection kit and then you go and meet your cadaver,' orders Joan.

All the students dash to make a queue. I am last because it takes me longer to get there. I feel awkward and frustrated but Alison stays alongside me. While we are in the queue we chat about our homes and schools. They seem so far away now and we feel very grown-up.

'Are you going to the initiation ceremony tonight?' she asks.

'Of course! I thought we had to.'

'Well, anybody who doesn't go isn't a proper Liverpool medic. It gets quite rough, apparently.'

I look at her, worried again. I am wondering how I will manage with my cumbersome artificial leg and crutches. There are so many little practical problems I hadn't thought about. However, the initiation ceremony is famous, not just in Liverpool but throughout the entire med school world. All we know is that it is horrible but compulsory. I am quiet as I ponder the problem of undergoing it.

Then Alison interjects: 'Before the ceremony a group of us are going for supper at this trendy bistro we've discovered. Do you want to come along? Then we can all give you a hand and shield you from the ruffians!'

'That would be great!' I say happily as we reach Joan and Rita and collect our dissection equipment.

'This is the moment we've been waiting for,' I say as we surround the table. I am not quite sure what I expect to see – perhaps bodies with expressions of torment on their faces. The dissection tables are made of gleaming, shiny metal. On each one, a large bulky shape is covered with a heavy rubber cloth. The sharp smell of formalin is so overpowering that our eyes begin to smart. A young doctor in a white coat issues us with instructions. We learn he is training to be a surgeon and is called a demonstrator. He is on hand if we become stuck.

'Fold back your cadaver covers, turn to page one in the manual – and then begin.'

Quickly we introduce ourselves to the rest of the table.

'I'm Alison, this is Mary. We'll take the left half.'

'I'm Helen and this is Ruth. We're fine with the right half.'

'Okay – so who is going to pull the cover back?' asks Alison. We all stand there looking at each other. All the tables are having the same dilemma. In a moment of bravery and with an over-enthusiastic desire to be accepted, I volunteer. I have to prove myself; I don't want any allowances made for me because of my leg.

'I'll do it.'

I have heard and faced death. I may as well look at it. Carefully I don disposable gloves and pull back the heavy cover.

The cadaver is lying face down and looks totally inhuman. It is cold and white and beached. I feel no emotion as I look at it, only an insatiable curiosity. I look carefully at the leg. In a few weeks I will have to cut into its dead skin. How will I cope with that? I think about my own leg and fleetingly I wonder what became of it. I push the thought away – there is no time now. As I prod the cold and lifeless flesh I remember my vow to survive. I shall not become a dead body on a cold metal table.

My new friends look at me with respect. 'It's fine,' I say. 'It just feels like putty.'

'Roll it to one side, Mary,' says Alison. 'The first thing we need to know is what sex it is.' We all giggle.

'Here goes then … flip, it weighs a ton,' I say. 'I could do with a hand.'

Helen snorts with laughter. 'Do you want the left or the right?' And we all burst into fits of giggles again.

'Man!' I announce, and let him drop back on the table with a heavy thud.

'Well, make the first cut, then,' says Alison, handing me the knife.

I take it from her and look at it carefully and slowly. I think back to the time at school when we cut into the rat. Back then, I kept thinking about Mr Peach cutting into my leg. This time it is a real human body. I think of all the times I wanted to cut into my own body to empty myself of the pain. My heart beats fast and I feel sweaty and clammy. I swallow hard. I need to do this. I have to be able to dissect the body if I am to remain at medical school. I think of the pride in my dad's face when he gave me his own dissection kit. I think of Mr Peach and his obvious delight when I went to tell him I was going to medical school.

'I'm so proud of you, Little Lady!' he said, and clapped me on the back so hard I nearly lost my balance.

I look around at the expectant faces of my fellow students. Inside, I feel a huge rush of courage. I am going to do this for my dad, for Mr Peach and for Dr Jimmy. I am here and I am going to make the first incision. Nobody ever expected I would see this day and I intend to live med school to the full because next term, even next week, is not guaranteed. I may never read chapter two of the dissection manual.

'Where do I start?' I ask.

Once dissection practical is over, Joan and Rita, who are obviously a double-act, show us to a large lecture room. It is filled with bones. Skeletons hang from large hooks. The walls are covered with posters of joints and muscles. There are square pots on shelves with pathology specimens inside. My eyes are drawn to one. It is a shaft of bone with a large lump attached to it and my heart lurches as I realize it is a Limpet. Filled with morbid curiosity, I take a closer look. It is labelled 'Osteogenic sarcoma of femur'. I remember its medical name as it was written down on my notes.

I peer at the killer Limpet. It is cut in half. I feel a gloating sense of victory that a Limpet is stuck in a pot of poisonous formalin, captured and exposed for ever. I can see its inside. It is a mixture of bone and bloody marrow. Its innocent appearance belies its deadly, horrible nature. I see how tightly it is fixed and, underneath, the tentacles of bad cells invading the healthy bone, streaking dark and ugly within the marrow. At last I am confronting my enemy. Perhaps my own Limpet is stuck in a pot somewhere, forever trapped as a punishment for taking my leg.

Alison looks over my shoulder curiously. 'What are you looking at?'

'The enemy. It's an osteosarcoma. That's the type of cancer I had.'

'Let me see,' and she picks up the pot to look more closely.

Mentally I spit at the tumour as I feel tears pricking my eyes. She pulls at my sleeve. 'Come on, leave the enemy there. We need to collect our skeletons.'

I part company with Alison outside the anatomy building. I am alone. We have arranged to meet up later for supper but now I need to get back to halls and dump my heavy skeletal friend. My skeleton is female. She is disassembled and her home is a large rectangular cardboard box. I am one of the last students out of the building. I didn't want to use the lift in front of all my new friends, so I walked painfully and slowly down the stairs from the anatomy lab. By that time the other students were long gone.

Now I am left standing in Ashton Street. I need to walk up a steep hill to the bus stop. Alison has put the box on the floor for me. Of course, she has not realized how difficult it is for me to carry stuff on my crutches. I was too proud to ask her for any more help and now I contemplate the dilemma I am in. Last night in my bright and cheerful room I prayed God would send me a helpmate. It is so difficult just getting around – and that is before my studies begin. I quickly utter another half-hearted prayer and wait. After a few minutes nobody arrives and I look impatiently at my watch. I realize that if I don't hurry I will miss the last bus back to halls. I will just have to solve the problem myself. I am filled with frustration as I contemplate how to carry the heavy box while using my crutches.

Sometimes I use a single crutch for short distances. I look ahead, measuring the long steep hill. But then what will I do with the other crutch? I can't leave it here because I will need it tonight at the initiation ceremony.

I place the left crutch on the handle of the right one. Then I put my hand over both crutches. So far, so good. Then I bend down and try to pick up the box with my other hand. After much heaving and panting I manage to trap the box between my hand and my artificial leg and I laboriously manoeuvre the box up my left side until it is tucked under my arm. It is not very well balanced but I squeeze it tightly against my body.

'Please, God, don't let me fall,' I pray. Experimentally, I take a few steps. It seems to work. I take a few more paces. But now I can feel the box sliding backwards so I stop and tighten my grip. This is going to take ages, I can see, and I worry again about missing the bus. So I try to walk a little more quickly. Suddenly the whole box slides backwards.

'Oh, no!' I shout, as it falls to the floor. To my horror, the precious bones of my unnamed female friend spill on to the pavement where they lie in a gruesome heap.

'Stupid, stupid thing!' I yell to the silence as my eyes begin to fill up. Now I will miss the bus. I am stranded and I have no idea how I will get to the supper venue or the initiation ceremony. 'Stupid leg! It wrecks everything! Why does it have to be me, God? It just isn't fair!' I fume under my breath.

Suddenly I hear a cheerful voice behind me. 'May I assist you with your skeleton?'

I turn to see a handsome young medical student grinning at me. He is also carrying a skeleton box and he obviously finds my predicament very amusing. I contemplate yelling at him to go away but then realize I am not in a very strong position.

'Oh, thank heavens!' I smile sweetly at him. 'You arrived at just the right moment, as you can see.'

'Well, I hope there aren't any broken bones!' He puts his own box on the floor and picks up my female friend, restoring her to her cardboard home. 'What on earth were you doing anyway?' he says, as I sort my crutches out and re-gather my thoughts and my dignity.

'What does it look like? I was trying to carry the box up the hill to the bus stop but these stupid crutches get in the way!' I am not in the mood for wisecracks.

'Why are you using crutches? I noticed you in the lab but didn't get a chance to talk to you. What's wrong with your leg?'

I reply crossly: 'Nothing – I haven't got one.' There are a few moments' silence as my new companion takes this in and picks up both skeletons. I wonder what he will say next.

'Well, I'm Richard Self and I'm going back to halls. Where are you going?'

'Dale Hall. I'm Mary Clewlow and I'm sorry for being cross but it's been rather a long day.'

'Well, we're heading the same way, so come on or we'll miss the bus.' He smiles easily at me and I decide I like him after all.

Suddenly a thought pops into my head from nowhere. It says: 'I've chosen him for you.'

As we sit on the bus we chat about the day.

'How come you were so late getting out of the anatomy building?' I ask. I look more closely at him. He has a crop of sandy hair and piercing blue eyes. I guess he is probably about six foot tall. I decide he is very good-looking.

'I was looking around the lab with the bones and pathology pots. There were some fabulous things to see. There's even a pot with Siamese twins in it.'

I fall silent as I remember the pot with the Limpet.

'My bone tumour is in that lab. It's called an osteogenic sarcoma.'

'So that's how you lost your leg, then?'

'Yep. I call it the Limpet. That's what it looks like.'

'How are you now? Are you okay?'

'Well, yes. I still have to go for check-ups.'

'What's your prognosis now, then? You don't mind me asking, do you?'

'Well, not that good. My dad is a doctor and in his book it says that only five per cent of people who have this tumour survive two years.'

Richard looks shocked and his face pales.

'I shouldn't really have opened my dad's book,' I explain. 'He said I wasn't allowed to read that one. But one night I looked it up.'

'Didn't the doctors tell you anything, though?'

'No, not really. Not at Christie's. At least not that I can remember. I was pretty ill after the chemotherapy. My hair fell out – can you tell?'

'No, I just thought maybe you liked short hair. I think your hair looks cute.'

'Yes, that's what Barry says – he's my boyfriend.'

'Well, my girlfriend has long hair, but I prefer short hair really.' There is an awkward silence as we both think about our friends back home.

'So is your dad a surgeon, then?'

'No, he's a general practitioner. The book was from when he was training, I guess.'

'But that must be ages ago. How old was the book?'

'Oh pretty old, I'd say. Why?'

'Well, it's probably out of date. I mean, they only just discovered chemotherapy recently, didn't they? That changes the outlook. Your dad's book would have been written maybe even before radiotherapy.'

'I never even thought of that. I remember Dad saying the chemo drugs were pretty new – and I had a new type of chemo!'

'What we need to do is find something more up-to-date. That would give us a better idea of your outlook.'

'Where would we find that?'

'We're medical students now. There are thousands of books and papers. We can read about any medical condition we want.'

'So maybe my outlook is better than I thought …'

'I'm sure it must be; it stands to reason. Chemotherapy must improve it, or what would be the point in using it? Tell you what, I'll go on a search and find out for you. I'll do it tomorrow – first lecture break.'

'Thank you! You don't know how much it means to me.'

'That's okay,' and he smiles. 'But you've just promised me the first dance at the freshers' party tonight.'

'It's a deal!' We smile broadly at each other and my heart skips a beat.

Richard helps me carry my skeleton up to my room and we part company, promising to meet at the dance.

I prepare for the evening ahead and think about all that has happened to me today. It has been exciting but I cannot remember being so tired. I have walked further than ever before since my amputation. My Little Leg is hurting and I have a whole evening ahead. I sink into my big beanbag, remove my artificial leg and throw it into a corner. My Little Leg is bruised and sore from the long hours on my feet and my phantom pains have re-started. Slowly I sigh and a wave of depression sweeps over me. How on earth am I going to get through the first week, let alone the first term? What if my Little Leg breaks down? Mr Peach and John Jackett are always warning me about that. My hip graft is rubbed and tender, too, and I ache all over. Tonight is the initiation ceremony and I also have to read up the dissection I have done today.

I am lost in my moody thoughts when there is a knock on the door.

'Hi! Can I come in? I'm Judith and we're in the same corridor. I'm a medic too.'

'Sure – I hope you don't mind, though. I'm an amputee and my leg is over there, so I can't get up.'

'That's okay,' she says, appearing unconcerned at my strange welcome. 'I've just come back from Lourdes. I looked after a couple of recent amputees there so I'm quite used to artificial legs all over the place.'

'What a coincidence! I went there, too, over the summer. I went on this pilgrimage to ask to be healed from my bone cancer.'

'Well, I went over to work as a handmaid in the hospital.'

We swop stories about our homes, schools and faiths.

'So do you just go to church,' asks Judith, 'or have you made a Christian commitment? You know – asked Jesus into your life?'

'Yes, I have. I did it just before I got ill.'

'Me too!' We beam at each other as we discover how much we have in common. I explain to Judith about the problems with my Little Leg and my phantom pains and tell her about my worries.

'I just don't know how I'm going to cope,' I finish.

'Well, you've two choices as I see it. Go home and come back next year … or stay and we'll help you all we can.'

'I can't go home and come back next year. I might not be here. What if my cancer relapses? I'm still going back to Christie's every two weeks.'

'Then you have no choice. Stay – fight – survive!' Judith gives me a hug. 'Come on, get your leg on. We can share a taxi. By the way, does your leg have a name?' She picks it up and hands it to me. 'It weighs a ton, Mary. No wonder you feel so tired.'

It actually weighs about half a stone.

'A name? For my leg? No, I've never thought of that!'

'We should give it a name. How about … Lee-Roy! After that dancer from the TV programme, *Fame!*'

'You're crazy!' I joke and shake my head. Her cheerful optimism is infectious. 'Okay, Lee-Roy he is!'

After a bistro supper with Alison and Judith plus a whole gang of other medics, we make our way nervously to the Old Lecture Theatre where the initiation ceremony takes place. Alison signals to Big John. 'Stay by us!' she orders him. 'You're in charge of Mary!'

We make our way on stage and the lights are switched off. The room is completely blacked out and we all wait. The entire medical school is gathered. We are suddenly pelted with all sorts of different objects – some smelly, some messy and some sticky. Paint, ketchup and rotten eggs are thrown at us from all directions, followed by feathers and flour. The stage is soon covered in a sea of mess. Then out come the hoses and we are sprayed liberally with freezing cold water!

As Judith and I change into clean clothes for the dance we cannot stop laughing.

'Have you decided whether you are going home, then?' she asks me playfully.

'I can't, can I? I need to get my own back – next year!'

I look at Judith with a sense of shock. 'Oh no, I said it!'

'Said what?'

'Next year … I never say that, just in case the sword falls.'

'Hey,' says Judith sternly. 'It's not going to fall. We are both going to be doctors, Mary, okay?'

Later, at the party, I find Richard and we compare horror stories about the initiation ceremony.

I abandon my crutches and we get up to dance to a Roxy Music number. Richard grabs my hand as we walk across the dance floor and pulls me to face him. For a moment I think he is going to kiss me as he holds my face in his hands, but he doesn't. He just smiles at me and looks closely into my eyes.

'Can you believe you're here?' he says.

'No, Richard, I honestly can't,' I reply. And it's true – I cannot believe

I am here at medical school, alive, laughing and looking into the eyes of a man with whom I am already falling in love.

'Well, Dr Clewlow-to-be, neither can I.' Then he adds, 'Did anyone ever tell you that you have the most amazing eyes?'

'Funnily enough, Dr Self-to-be ... no! You're the first person ever to tell me that.'

We dance, with a little help from Lee-Roy, and that most awful day in January when I asked Mr Peach if I could ever be a doctor seems a long, long time ago.

The next day Richard seeks me out at lunchtime. Judith and I are sitting together in the medical students' common room.

'I've been to the library for you. I just wanted to let you know that I'm still working on it but it's quite rare, this tumour, isn't it? It might take me a few weeks to find everything. But I haven't forgotten.'

'Thanks, Richard.'

'Too bad he's already taken,' says Judith.

'I know he has a girlfriend back home.'

'Yes – really serious thing, apparently. Been together for ages and desperately in love and all that.'

'Oh. I kind of had the impression it wasn't like that.'

'Why? You sound disappointed. Do you like him?'

'No,' I say defensively. 'I mean, I like him, but I've got a boyfriend at home anyway.' I tell her about Barry and wonder what he would make of this strange world in which, even after such a short space of time, I am already totally immersed.

'I don't think it will last, really,' I sigh, and look at my friend. 'I don't know if it's all that fair, anyway. I mean, I'll be here for five years. What kind of chance will it stand? It isn't just that, either. He is part of my illness. I think I need a new life – you know, put that bit of my life away. He will always be part of being so desperately sick.'

That night I write to Barry and explain about my new life and moving on. I feel guilty as I tearfully post it because his friendship helped me get through the summer. Every morning I check my mail for a reply but nothing arrives.

As the days pass, full of lectures and practicals, my letters home recount the tales of my new life. I bury the memories and the days of despair. I paint over the fear and the pain. As I recovered from the chemotherapy, my A levels absorbed me. Now medicine becomes my learning challenge. I fill my hours with bones, joints and muscles. I am learning, too, about living and laughing again as I make new friends and build a fresh store of experiences.

But at night, lying in my room, my thoughts return to the Limpet. I picture the evil cells streaking into the bone marrow in the pathology specimen and shudder. I still follow a routine of checking my body for the offspring of the Limpet. I start with my good leg and check the smooth contours. Then I feel all over my abdomen and move up to my breasts and arms. I feel under my armpits and then around my neck. There is nothing I can do about checking my brain, but I guess I would know pretty soon if I had a metastasis there. Lumps – that's what I am looking for. Limpet lumps. And then I begin the day knowing that today there are none. I'm clear.

A few weeks into term, I have to return to Christie's for a check-up. It is the first time since starting med school and I am deep in thought in the common room, feeling depressed at the prospect, when Big John comes over.

'Why are you looking so miserable?'

'I have to go back to Christie's today. I'm worrying about it. I'm so frightened of that place. Even the thought of it makes me terrified.'

'Are you going alone?'

'Yes, I'm meeting my dad there.'

'Well, I'll tell you what. How about if I come with you? My home's not far from Christie's and I can make a surprise visit. We could catch the train together and I'll escort you to wherever you're meeting your dad.'

Big John has become my main piggy-back provider. Friday mornings he meets me out of histology lectures and carries me over to the organic chemistry building while one of the other lads takes my crutches. It is about half a mile but he doesn't seem to notice my weight. He just says: 'Good rugby training!' It is part of what has become a very happy formula. Big John piggy-backs me; Alison makes sure I don't have to stand up for too long in dissection; Judith helps me get around in hall and when I have a bath and Richard looks after me on the bus. Sometimes I feel awkward about needing help and I squirm inside when I can't do the things I used to be able to do, but I am learning to control my frustration.

Big John and I agree the trip to Manchester and he makes sure I arrive safely.

'You'll be fine – I'll see you later and you can tell me the good news.'

I walk slowly through the front doors I passed through when I first came here back in February. Then I was lying on a stretcher: now I am walking on Lee-Roy, using a single crutch to help me. Back then I couldn't even balance. Now I can stand steadily enough to dissect out veins and nerves. I recollect how strange medical words seemed to me then, and now they are part of my everyday conversation. I am learning about femurs and drugs. I now know how to spell osteogenic sarcoma.

As I enter the hospital the astringent antiseptic smell is no longer foreign. It has become part of the air I breathe. And yet my heart begins to beat faster. I walk past the signs to the CT scan and the isotope room and I feel hot and sweaty. I am early and cannot think of waiting in the clinic, so I head along the corridor to Ward Two. The route is so familiar, the corridor wide with green swirly tiles. Here and there are abandoned trolleys. I stop outside, faltering, my mouth dry. My palms are moist and I rub them on my combat trousers. Although I have revisited Christie's many times for my check-ups, I have never made this trip back to Ward Two. I spot Vera through the door window, bustling to and fro, and smile as I push the door and greet her.

'Mary! It's our own Dr Mary!' she calls, and Sister Anna comes out of the office.

'Hey, I've a long way to go before you can call me doctor!' I say as they fuss round me, asking dozens of questions about my studies and medical school.

'Do you want to come and see old Edith?' asks Vera, referring to the bed I slept in.

'I'm not sure ...'

'Come on – it will do you good to see how far you've come in such a short time. We don't get many patients coming back as medical students!'

I am not prepared for the rush of emotion I feel when I see the bed. The notice is still there, the brass still shining. 'Edith Cavell bed', I read under my breath. A middle-aged lady, sitting on it, is completely bald. Self-consciously she puts a hand to her scalp.

'It's okay,' I say, much more cheerfully than I feel. 'My hair fell out too – I know how you feel.' The lady smiles at me, admiring my thick crop of curls.

'Was your hair so curly before?' she asks.

I shake my head. 'No – more or less straight. Your hair may grow back differently. That's because of the way the drugs affect the cells of your scalp.'

The lady looks at me, amazed. 'Well, I'm so glad to have met you. I was feeling really down about my hair.'

As we walk up the ward together Vera whispers to me: 'That's why I wanted you to meet Edith!' We smile knowingly. It feels so good to be able to bring a bit of hope back into the ward.

'Are you off to the chapel, then?' asks Vera as I leave.

'Yes, I think I will go up. I've still got half an hour to kill.'

The rubbery smell in the lift makes me recall vividly the last journey I made up here. I shake my head slowly as I remember the tears I shed. My heart begins to race again as I enter the small room. It is like walking back in time. Everything seems untouched since my last visit. The tapestry of the Last Supper hangs above the altar, only this time the figures are very definitely stitched to the canvas. The dilemma I struggled with in this place has gone. I shall never side with Judas. Leaving the chapel, I close the door firmly and quietly. I shall not return here again, ever. It reminds me of despair. And now the door is for ever closed on despair.

A little later I have my check-up and am told I am clear. I have beaten the Limpet for another round and I have a new doctor, too. From now on my care will be overseen by Dr Gupta, a small, smiling and efficient consultant oncologist. I am also told I will be able to see him at the Victoria Hospital in my home town of Blackpool and will not need to return to Christie's.

I meet Big John at the hospital gates, and he lifts me up and gives me a huge hug to celebrate. 'Looks like you get to sit the Christmas exams!'

So I make that my next goal and study hard. I make it to the exams – I make it to Christmas – and before I know it I am home with my family again.

'Is it okay if one of my friends visits over New Year?' I ask my parents.

'Of course,' they agree, and ask who it will be.

'Oh, one of the boys from our year,' and I see my mum and dad exchange glances.

I try to conceal my excitement about my new boyfriend. 'Actually, we're going out together. You'll like him. He's called Richard.' I smile secretively and head up to my bedroom where I daydream about the new man in my life.

It all began when he told me about the research he had done on my tumour. One day he came over with loads of medical papers.

'It's good news, really.'

'Tell me! Hurry up!'

'Well, with your regime, the five-year survival rate is between twenty-five and forty per cent. That means you have a forty per cent chance of surviving five years, if you believe the most favourable studies.'

'That is much better than I thought possible. I mean, that's a pretty good chance, really.'

'The other thing I found out is that most people who don't make it tend to die in the first two years.'

'Well, I'm almost at one year since my illness was discovered, so I'm halfway through!'

'Precisely!' We both laughed and I shook my head again.

'I can't believe it. Thank you so much.'

It seemed appropriate that we were sitting in the medical school common room which had been decked festively for the approaching Christmas party.

'I was thinking, too – would you like to come to the Christmas dance with me tomorrow? We can celebrate your good news!'

'I'd love to,' I said, as nonchalantly as I could when, in truth, my heart was racing!

We danced and had a good time and then somebody produced the mistletoe and now we are going out together. He is coming over on New Year's Eve to help me take my mind off the first anniversary of my operation …

I sing 'Auld Lang Syne' surrounded by my family and Richard. I see in the New Year of 1984 with a kiss. I think back to the last time I heard the words of the song and shudder. And I am unprepared for how I am hit again by the pain of loss as I reach 7 January. It is a whole year since my leg was amputated and my life changed for ever. As soon as I open my eyes the day looms ahead of me, a chasm of dark and depressing thoughts. I wander down to join my friends for breakfast at the beginning of the new term and check my mail box. Rolled up inside is a poster with a message from Richard.

I unwrap my gift and read the words carefully: 'Keep your face to the sunshine and you will not see the shadows.' I smile and fix the poster on my wall, promising myself I will put it up on every anniversary I reach.

Later we meet at lectures.

'How shall we spend your first anniversary?'

'Let's go somewhere new. I don't feel like sitting in lectures today. I don't think I could concentrate.'

'I have the perfect plan.' Richard looks at me. 'We'll see Liverpool from its best vantage point.'

So we take a bus down to the Pier Head. It is bright, cold and windy. Richard points out the beautiful buildings of the waterfront one by one.

'Let's catch a ferry,' he suggests, and scoops me up and piggy-backs me down the steep ramp. We lean over the sides, watching the murky waters of the River Mersey flow past.

'Sing one of your Beatles numbers?' Richard asks.

I climb on a bench and strike up with a favourite: 'Eight Days a Week'. As I jump off the bench into his arms he holds me tight and kisses me.

'I'll share every anniversary. I'll be here every year for you,' he tells me as he looks deeply into my eyes. 'I love you, Mary Clewlow.'

'I love you, too ...'

My second anniversary brings with it the prospect of my second Bachelor of Medicine exams. After finals, they are the most important in medical school. They include anatomy, physiology and biochemistry – the foundations of medicine. By the end of our anatomy course we complete dissecting our cadaver. The worst bit, of course, is cutting up the leg. Alison knows it will be difficult for me so she does the first incision. It is all right until we get to the point where we have to remove the leg from the body in order to discover how the hip joint works.

'I'm not sure I can do this bit, Alison,' I tell my friend. 'It's too close to what I went through.'

'Don't worry,' she reassures me, 'you read out the manual and I'll do the dissection.'

So we work as a team. Alison severs all the muscles which hold the leg in the hip joint. It is so strange watching her and thinking what must have happened during my operation. Then comes the point where we need to take the leg away from the body.

'You hold the leg, Mary,' she says, 'while I dislocate it.'

So I hold the leg and Alison works slowly but methodically.

'Pull,' she says.

Suddenly the leg comes away from the body and I am left holding it in my arms. 'Oh help, Alison. I think I'm going to faint.'

I have this severed leg in my arms and nowhere to put it. I cannot let go of it. It is as if I am rooted to the spot. All I can think is that some-body – a nurse maybe – held my leg in exactly the same way. Were they surprised by the dead weight of it, as I am?

'Mary, put the leg down,' I hear Alison's voice echoing around my head.

'What happened to mine?' I suddenly realize I have no idea what became of my lost left leg.

'Mary, come on, I've made a space here. Now put it down for good-ness sake before you drop it on the floor.'

I laugh a harsh and empty laugh. It feels like hysteria. The leg is cold and heavy and stiff. It is very dead. I think, with a shock, that my leg would not have been cold and lifeless – it would have been warm and bloody. Alison gently takes the leg from me and leads me over to a stool. She fetches Joan and Rita who take me to the common room and give me a cup of tea. Joan puts her arms around me as I weep from the shock of it all.

'I just kept wondering what became of my leg,' I explain to her. 'That's why I was upset. It wasn't the actual dissection.'

'Well, why don't you ask somebody? Then you'll know for sure. How about if I ask one of the demonstrators to come and tell you? They are all surgeons. They would know.'

So Joan has a chat with one of the kinder demonstrators. He tells me what would have happened to my leg.

'First, they would have taken a lot of it, including the tumour, for pathology tests, to diagnose the cancer.'

'How would they have done that?'

'By softening the bone tumour, slicing it up and making it into microscope slides.'

'So it isn't in a pot, then?'

'No, it will be on slides and kept safely just in case they ever need to check it again.'

'And the rest of it?'

He looks at me cautiously. 'Well … the rest of the leg would have been put in a big yellow bag. Then it would have been taken for disposal.'

'And how do they do that?'

There is a silence. He looks horrified.

'I need to know. Not knowing is worse. I've never had to think about it before. It's going round and round in my head, thinking about where my left leg is.'

'It would have been burnt.'

So, finally, I know.

'Kind of cremated?'

'Exactly.'

Joan squeezes my hand in support.

'In fact,' Mark adds, 'in previous times, if somebody lost a limb it would be buried … given a sort of funeral service. Maybe that would be helpful for you to know.'

'Yes, it is.'

Later on, Judith, Richard and I meet up in the chapel. We hold a final service of farewell for my amputated leg which, as I now know, was cremated two years earlier. We read some scripture and Judith plays 'Be not afraid' on her guitar. That day I reach a watershed in my life; I bury my left leg for ever.

With the passing of my second anniversary there is much to celebrate. Dr Gupta spells out the significance.

'Mary, it's great news that your tests are clear today. Two years is very important with your type of cancer. You know now that osteosarcoma relapses early. Nearly always in the first two years. This is a big milestone.'

'I know, Dr Gupta. Ninety-five per cent of patients who relapse do so in the first two years. So things are looking good, yes?'

'Indeed they are. How are you going to celebrate?'

'I can't celebrate! I've got my second MB in a few weeks. I have so much revision to do. I'll have to delay the celebration until afterwards!'

'And then,' laughs Dr Gupta, 'you get to meet real patients!'

During the clinical years, medical students are arranged into small groups of about six. The group is called a 'firm' and usually stays together. My firm includes Richard, Judith, Alison and John Wakefield, whom we call JW. The first clinical attachment is in general surgery. On our first day we gather, wearing our brand new, pristine white coats. Our pockets are bulging with stethoscopes, notebooks and tourniquets. We have listened to lectures on how to take case histories and practised clinical examination on each other but today it is for real. Soon we meet the consultant on our firm, Mr Sells. He is tall, dark and distinguished and we are all absolutely terrified of him. He demands perfection. We are given a list of first-ever real patients to see, and nervously we approach them. Mine is an elderly man with a very strong Scouse accent. I take out my notebook and pen and prepare to ask my first question. I have rehearsed this moment many times.

'So then, what brought you to hospital?'

I wait with baited breath for my first-ever patient to answer.

'An ambulance, queen.'

The next question dies on my lips as I blush deeply and the nurse making the bed opposite giggles.

'She means, what's wrong with you, Charlie?'

'Oh, it's this,' he says. Casting aside the bed cover, he pulls down his pyjamas to reveal a hugely swollen testicle. 'Here you are, queen, you can feel it, too. Everybody else on this bloody ward has. I'll be charging soon.'

This is my grand introduction to clinical medicine. Since then I have lost count of the number of patients I have seen and the number of fierce consultants in front of whom I have blushed. Being a medical student is great, but at times life is a bit humiliating. Just when you think you're beginning to get somewhere, something happens to make you see how much there is to learn. Even the student nurses seem to get a better deal – at least they make a practical contribution, whereas we are just seen as getting in the way.

I soon come face to face with my first cancer patient. It is really hard. She is middle-aged, with breast cancer. She has already had a biopsy and needs to have her breast removed. I feel so nervous when I sit down beside her. I ask the routine questions: 'When did you find the lump?' 'Did you have any pain …?'

'I'm just so scared of the cancer,' she confesses. 'I mean, it's hard enough to think about losing my breast … but then I have to worry about whether or not I will make it.'

I don't reply – I am in my own world, running parallel with hers.

'I can't bear to think how my body will be so different. I keep wondering if I will still be loved with only one breast.'

I am struggling to hold back the tears but I know I have to keep control.

'Then I need to have chemotherapy and I'm scared about that, too. I'll lose my hair, they say. It all seems so very frightening.'

'Yes,' I say without thinking, 'it is. Very frightening.'

The lady looks at me in surprise. 'Oh! You're the first person who has understood. Thank you.'

I smile at her. It feels so good to hear those words. For the first time, I feel it is true about things being for a purpose. After that, I adore every minute of my clinical studies. I love being on the wards, seeing patients, helping in the operating theatre and casualty. I love just being there, chatting to the nurses and soaking up the atmosphere. It is hard work and there are days when I get home, throw my leg into a corner, soak in a bath and sleep. I get so tired – but it is worth it to see that look of surprise and hear the words 'You seem to understand.' I now know that Mr Peach was definitely right when he said my experiences would make me a better doctor. For the first time since my operation, I don't feel at a disadvantage. In fact, sometimes I now think I wouldn't change places with my fellow students.

On the third anniversary I am approaching my twenty-first birthday – and how different it feels from the year I celebrated my eighteenth. Now I've done lots of things I never imagined possible. Reaching my third anniversary I still believe in God, and I go to church sometimes, but really I have drifted away from the faith I once knew. When I look round the hospitals and see so much suffering I just cannot accept that a loving God could allow such terrible pain.

About this time, our friends around us are settling down in steady relationships. Some become engaged and others move in together. Richard and I are counted among the 'steadies'. As usual, we celebrate my anniversary together. We take a long walk up a hillside in Cheshire. At the top we find an old ruined castle with a deep, deep well.

'If you could wish anything,' Richard asks me, 'would you wish your leg back?'

'Not any more. I used to, all the time. I guess now I know it doesn't stop me doing anything I want to. The hardest thing is coping with feeling different.'

'But being different is what makes you so beautiful.'

'Do you really think that? I get worried you won't like my body … I guess that's why I haven't felt ready to …'

'Oh, so that's the reason, is it? I thought it was your Catholic conscience. Well, for the record, I love you and I love your body.'

'But I think I look ugly and weird with only one leg.'

'Well, I don't and neither do any of your other dozen or so admirers.' We laugh together. 'Your body is just different. You sometimes look like a little mermaid sitting all curled up.'

I blush and smile again.

'So … do you think we should?'

We look at each other and giggle.

'Yes, I think we should,' I reply, and we walk hand in hand back down the hillside.

That night I undress in front of Richard. I show him my body and it is strange because I don't feel damaged or mutilated as I thought I would. I feel special and loved. The moment I have always dreaded – revealing my naked body to my lover – is truly wonderful. He doesn't mind my Little Leg being only little and he kisses my scars. Then we make love and somehow it seems as if I have always known it would be him. Thereafter, I guess I accept my body in a way I could not have imagined. I'm not ugly – I'm just me.

My fourth anniversary brings with it dark shadows again – only this time they are following someone else. I arrive home from lectures to find a note pushed under my door.

'Dear Mary,' it reads, 'there is a first-year medic who would love to meet you. She is called Sara and is in the intensive care unit at the Royal Liverpool Hospital. I'm sure you could help her.' It is signed by one of the medics in our year.

I know the story of Sara – the entire medical school has heard how a first-year student contracted meningitis, suffered failure of all her body organs and underwent amputation of both legs. I assumed she had died. I sit down and re-read the letter. So many feelings come flooding back. I remember the loss of my own leg. It is hard to imagine how it must feel to wake from an illness to discover you have lost both.

I also remember lying in bed every morning, slowly opening my eyes and praying my leg had grown back. Now I know lots of amputees feel like that – it is all part of denying the loss.

'I don't know whether I am up to this,' I say to Richard later.

'Well, if you aren't then I don't know anybody who is.'

'But what do I say to her? I've never really got involved with anybody else who has lost a limb.'

'Tell her what you would have wanted to hear. What bothered you the most?'

'What my new body would look like. I was scared of the mutilation.'

'Well, go and show her how attractive you are, then. Put on your trendiest gear and knock the socks off the intensive care unit.'

So I do. I dress up in one of my short kilts. John Jackett has made me a new leg using the latest technology and poor old Lee-Roy is now consigned to a cupboard. This new leg is lightweight and rather shapely. In fact, with a little ingenuity, I can wear mini-skirts with no problem.

As I ring the bell to enter Intensive Care I feel very nervous. I want so much to bring hope to Sara. A nurse shows me into a tiny waiting room.

'This is Sara's mum. I'll leave you two together.'

Margaret comes over and throws her arms around me.

'You don't know how much this means to us,' she cries. 'Look at you! I can't even tell you're an amputee. And you're wearing such fashionable clothes.'

We sit down and Margaret tells me her daughter's story.

'She rang one night to say she had a headache and was going to bed. The next day we received a call to say she was dangerously ill.' She goes on to tell me how the doctors almost gave up hope.

'Everybody prayed – we are Christians, you see – and she pulled through. The doctors said it was incredible … but then her legs lost circulation and we had to make the decision whether to lose her or agree to the amputations. When Sara woke we had to tell her both her legs were gone below the knees.'

I listen with tears streaming down my face. 'I don't know what to say, Margaret. I can only imagine a fraction of what you have all gone through.'

'Oh no,' says Margaret. 'You are the only one who will understand how Sara feels. Please go in and see her.'

And that's how I first met Sara. Now I visit her often. She always tells me how glad she was that I was wearing my trendy mini-skirt.

'I thought I would never be attractive again,' she says when we reminisce about that day. 'Then you walked into my room with your make-up and your mini-skirt. You hitched up your *very* short skirt and asked me which was the real leg – and I couldn't tell!'

I share lots of practical hints with her – what to wear and how to feel good about yourself. I tell her about Richard and how we have no problem with sex or anything like that. I tell her how to get around medical school and how to cope with the heavy hours. I tell her about learning to drive a car as soon as possible and regaining her independence.

In return, she tells me how her faith enables her to get through ... and something in me responds. It is hard to listen to Sara and ignore the effect Jesus has upon her life. So I begin to think about God again. Sometimes I even read my Bible and pray, like I used to. But throughout my student years my faith, once so solid, has been in a state of flux.

My final year at medical school brings a difficult hurdle. I begin my obstetrics course. I was dreading it because I knew I would be seeing tiny newborn babies all the time. I wasn't sure how I would feel. The results of the chemotherapy on my fertility are still unclear. Dr Gupta is evasive whenever I ask him.

'We don't know,' he says. 'But it's unlikely that your fertility is normal.'

So I have come to terms with not having children – until I do my obstetrics. The first delivery I watch is a young couple expecting their first child. I sit with them all the way through the labour and, to be honest, I don't expect to feel sad when the baby arrives. I thought I would feel excited at seeing my first birth. But, as I watch them holding their new baby daughter in their arms, I feel a huge pain in my heart. My arms ache to hold the baby. I want to make her the centre of my world, as she is of theirs. I feel so angry and cheated by God and once again I start to rant and rave at Him, blaming Him for everything I have lost because of the cancer. I turn my back on Him again, feeling it is so unnecessary to take my children in addition to my leg and perhaps my future.

The following day I have another shock when I sit with an older couple who are also waiting for their longed-for first child to arrive. The baby is in a breech position. I watch the delivery proceed but something starts to go wrong and the baby gets stuck. The midwives and doctors start to panic and I am asked to leave the room. I sit outside, praying with all my might for the baby to live. Everything goes crazy: doctors running in and out of the room, alarms sounding ... then a silence – a long, eerie silence. Next, I hear a scream of pain – the sound I made when I woke up from my amputation and discovered my leg was no more. It is a sound so full of mental and physical anguish that it makes the hairs stand up on the back of my neck. Immediately I recognize it as a cry of grief. I go back to my room, lie on the bed and weep. I weep for the babies I will never have. I weep for the loss of children I have never even thought about, let alone held. I weep for the lady in the tiny, joyless delivery room holding her dead baby. Then I recall the Romany boy running up to me all those years ago and I thump my pillow again and again.

'Lies,' I whisper. 'It's all stupid lies. There is no God, anyway.'

Heading towards my fifth anniversary, there seems to be a lot happening in my life once more. It is as if I am facing another crossroads. Medical finals are on the horizon. If I am successful, I will at last become Dr Mary Clewlow. Richard and I have been together more than four years now and we need to choose whether our futures are to be linked for ever. He has been here with me at every anniversary, as he promised. We have had our ups and downs but those landmarks we have always shared. In fact, we have shared everything. I have only made it here because of him. He has been my strong arm and my helpmate. As each anniversary passed and I stepped a little further away from the Limpet, I breathed another sigh of relief. I count not in years any more, but in anniversaries. When 7 January comes around, although I feel again the sadness of loss, I look up and see another safety net between me and the sword.

Now I am waiting for my friends to turn up to help me celebrate my fifth anniversary of being cancer-free. I needed to mark it with a party. It is the survival goal I have aimed for since Richard gave me the statistics. After five years the cancer can take a back seat in my life and after ten I can be discharged from medical care. This party is going to be special: a celebration of the vow, a celebration of my life surviving the Limpet. In fact, this is going to be the biggest party the medical school has ever seen.

It is 7 January 1988. Five whole years have passed since the day Mr Peach entered my room on Ward Eight and gave me the news that was to alter my life beyond recognition. In those five years I have lived and loved and laughed. I have known pain and fear and loss. But I have never given in to Judas. Despair has never won – and the Limpet is still at bay. Hundreds of my medical friends and family join the party. Our little student house is bursting at the seams. These are the comrades whose love and friendship has seen me through the last five years and their concern and joy for me is clearly genuine.

I am standing on a threshold. I am now one of the forty per cent. Behind me lies a path of uncertainty. The ghost of Damocles is still sitting in my place and the sword is still above my head, but I think I can now make some plans. I can begin to look ahead a little further. In the summer I will sit my finals. In a few short months it will be Easter, the time Richard and I have set to decide our future.

My friends and my family sing 'Congratulations' and we dance until the neighbours complain and the floorboards cave in. We are all dizzy with champagne and laughter. Hellie announces that I need to make a speech and Richard lifts me up onto the table with a glass of champagne in my hand.

I tell them: 'I only have one thing to say – it's the vow I made five years ago … I shall not die but I shall live.'

As I say the words to my audience, silence falls.

In my mind I hear an answer:

'I will lead you through.'

8

'Is that Dr Clewlow?' I ask, stifling my giggles, as my dad answers the surgery phone in his brisk, professional tone.

'Yes. Who's speaking?'

'This is Dr Clewlow, too!'

There is silence as my dad takes in the news.

'I passed my finals, Dad!'

I am laughing and dancing and fellow students in a lengthening queue for the public phone gesture to me impatiently. I hear my dad crying with pride and joy.

'I knew you would do it. I must ring your mum immediately. We are so proud of you.'

I walk over to where Richard is waiting and he puts his arms around me.

'I'm so proud of you, too!' He kisses me and takes hold of my left hand.

My emerald engagement ring catches the light and I smile again as I admire it.

'Well, I've decided that I will be Dr Clewlow this year and Dr Self next year.'

Richard looks surprised. 'Really? You mean you're going to practise under your married name and not your maiden name?'

'Yes, of course. It's too confusing having two Dr Clewlows.'

'Not as confusing as having two Dr Selfs in the same city!'

'Well, we can be him-Self and her-Self!'

He groans at the joke we have heard hundreds of times already. 'Come on, we have a ball to attend,' he urges, as we walk hand in hand up Ashton Street, where we first met five years ago.

'Do you remember the skeleton?' asks Richard.

'How could I forget? How foolish I must have looked! It seems so long ago now. I never imagined for a moment that I would reach this point. I never thought I would live to see this day.'

'Did you think we would end up engaged to be married?'

'Well … I've never told you this, but when I first met you I thought I heard somebody – presumably God – telling me you had been chosen for me. I thought at the time I was going crazy!'

'So when did you know we were meant for each other?'

'That's easy: my first cancer-free anniversary on the ferry … when I sang on the bench!'

'I knew it too – that's why I took you back there to ask you to marry me.'

I think back to the day Richard asked me to marry him as we walked up the familiar steep hill …

'Come on, I'm taking you on a surprise outing,' he said to me. It was a sharp, bright spring day, just before Easter 1988. Final exams were looming.

'Richard, I have so much work to do! I really need to finish this subject before tonight.' I turned back to my dull surgical textbook.

'No arguments. It's a beautiful sunny day. Wrap up warm, though.'

I put on my cosy duffel coat, wondering what Richard was planning. We headed towards the Pier Head. As we walked down the ferry ramp, the wind whipped round us.

'You have some crazy ideas!' I teased him. 'It will be freezing on the ferry!'

We settled ourselves out of the wind with cups of steaming hot chocolate and I watched the waves lapping around the boat.

'Come on, then, sing me one of your Beatles numbers. Remember, this is Liverpool!'

'Okay! Any requests?'

' "Eight days a week" – the first one you sang to me. Same bench, please!'

So I looked round for the original place. 'I think it was this one!'

I climbed up a lot more easily than I had done all those years before. I sang it and ended by leaping off the bench, laughing breathlessly. Richard caught and steadied me. Then, to my amazement, he got down on his knees.

'What are you doing? I wasn't that good!'

'I want to ask you something. Mary Clewlow – will you marry me?'

I was stunned. We had intended to talk about our future at Easter. He had caught me completely by surprise.

And so, looking at the skyline of our adopted city, I kissed Richard and became his fiancée. He dug into his pocket and produced a tiny box containing my ring – emerald and diamond, just perfect!

Later, we set the date for July the following year, 1989, and agreed to start wedding planning in earnest today – the day I qualify as a doctor.

'We need to begin making arrangements immediately,' I say to Richard. 'Once our house officer year gets under way we won't have a spare moment.'

'Do you want to get married in Blackpool?'

'No, I don't think so. Liverpool has become our home. I would like to get married here. This is where we have grown up together.'

I think for a few moments. 'I would like to get married in the Catholic cathedral with loads of family and all our colleagues. Then afterwards we should have a massive celebration.'

'Bridesmaids?'

'Franny, Hellie and Sara – she is almost a sister now.'

My friendship with Sara has strengthened since seeing her in hospital following her amputations. Now she is back in medical school and we share so many similar experiences.

'My best friend Alex can be best man, Judith and Adrian can do the music …'

'Well, I guess that's sorted! What a busy day – qualifying as a doctor and planning a wedding!' As we head home together to prepare for the graduation ball, I feel overwhelming joy to know I have survived the Limpet, am now a doctor and am also engaged to be married. I remember that first day in the anatomy lab when I stared angrily at the pickled Limpet. I laugh inside and cheer my victory.

The graduation ball is held at the Albert Docks in a ballroom decked with balloons and ribbons. Soon we are all flushed with whirling around and plenty of champagne. As the night draws to an end we gather for the prize-giving.

'Well, this won't bring any surprises,' we all say. One of our colleagues has won almost every prize there has ever been. Time after time his name is called out and we all tease him, pretending to stifle our yawns.

The Dean pauses. 'Now, the next prize is awarded for the highest mark in the clinical medicine exam. It's a real pleasure to award this to someone of whom we are all very proud … we have seen her overcome so much and win so many personal victories … she really has worked hard to achieve this – Dr Mary Clewlow!'

As I go forward to collect my prize I am crying with joy. All my fellow students cheer and applaud me loudly. I feel I am only here because of their support. I see Big John Kirwan waving and Alison is shouting out 'Well done!' As I arrive back at the table Richard kisses me and holds me tight. Without him I fear I would have given up long ago.

'I love you, Dr Mary Clewlow and Dr Mary Self-to-be!' he says, as he pulls me on to the dance floor again. And the dark clouds seem very, very far away.

I spend the summer planning the wedding and preparing for the arduous year ahead. Life as a house officer is gruelling and I need to be as mentally and physically fit as possible. My stubborn refusal to admit any limitation means I am going to be doing my house year full-time. There will not be much relaxing.

Richard and I spend time in the Lake District together and I raise a difficult subject. The sun is setting over the water at the end of a beautiful day. As ever, I have spent most of it in and out of the water, swimming in Lake Coniston. We huddle in layers of warm towels and blankets, sipping tea out of enamel mugs.

'Richard, I need to discuss something.'

'Mmm,' he replies, his mind elsewhere.

'It's about children.' I look down at the ground and start throwing stones into the lake. I feel the familiar anger rising. I still find it hard to accept that this pain was added to my cancer.

'You know – the chemotherapy and being infertile.'

'Yes, I know. You told me years ago about what the doctors said.'

'Well, I was thinking – if you want to change your mind, I'll understand.'

'What on earth do you mean?'

'About marrying me. If we can't have children – maybe you won't want to marry me.'

Richard stops what he is doing and crouches down beside me. He looks into my eyes and a tear rolls down my cheek. 'I find it so hard to contemplate – not holding my own baby in my arms. It's so unfair. I seem to have been through so much. Why has this been given to me as well?'

'I don't know. But you're alive. The chemotherapy saved your life. That's all that matters to me.'

'But I can't give you children.'

123

'That's not why I'm marrying you. I love you. It doesn't matter whether we have children or not. It's you I want.'

'Maybe you'll change your mind ...'

'Mary, I've always known about your cancer and your treatment. The research is still very uncertain in lots of areas. We've grown up with that. Nothing has ever been guaranteed. I still love you. I've always loved you and I always will. If we don't have children then we will fill our lives with other things. As long as I'm with you, that's all that matters.'

He wipes the tears from my face. 'Anyway, you believe in God. So do I – just about. When we get married, we'll pray for children – every day if you want. If we are meant to be parents then God will hear us.'

'For better or worse, remember?'

'Yes. In sickness and in health.'

We sit side by side, best friends till death us do part, and watch the lake darken. Only when we are shivering do we return home to Liverpool and the first day of our medical careers.

'Hello, I'm Dr Clewlow, the new house officer.'

It is 1 August 1988.

The sister barely looks at me before replying. 'Blood forms are there, IV drugs are waiting and Mr Cooke wants the operating list.'

Mr Cooke is the consultant for whom I am going to be working. He is a general surgeon at the Royal Liverpool Hospital.

I hardly have time to answer before the sister disappears. A staff nurse smiles at me.

'Hi, I'm Amanda. The room over there is where you will find everything to take your blood tests and the list of patients is here.' She points to a board and adds: 'Your patients are the ones written in green.' I seem to have by far the most.

'The blood porter arrives at ten, so do your bloods first or you'll miss him. Then go and find the secretary and submit your list. Then we'll do the intravenous drugs.'

She gives me an understanding smile.

'Don't worry, within a week you'll feel like you've been here for ever!'

I pick up the pile of blood forms and check the list left by the previous doctor. I look at my watch. It is already nine o'clock and I have at least an hour's worth of blood tests to take. At five past nine my newly acquired bleeper goes off. I am bleeped dozens of times in the space of half an hour. I fall behind with my routine work and miss the blood porter's round. The theatre list is submitted late and the morning's injections of intravenous drugs become lunchtime doses. Everybody shouts at me – from the theatre sister to the secretary. Now I understand Dr Jimmy's favourite moan: 'We're the lowest form of life on the ward.' I finish at 8.00 p.m. and drag myself home. I have not eaten all day. My head hurts, my Little Leg hurts, my foot hurts – in fact everything hurts! I must have walked miles today, just back and forth between departments. I lie on the bed and wonder how on earth I will get through this year.

Later I discuss my worries with Richard, who is working at the Walton Hospital in Liverpool. His day on the wards has been just as tiring, but he knows that physically I have been stretched to the limit.

'What am I going to do? I haven't even done my first on-call night yet!'

'How much do you want to get through this year?'

'You know how much it means to me. I have put everything into qualifying. I have to do my house year.'

'Right – you need to survive. Head down, grit teeth. You're a sticker and very stubborn. Make friends with the nurses. Get on the right side of all the people who can make life easier for you – the porters, the ward clerk, the secretary. It all cuts down on the things that are non-essential but which get dumped on us by default.'

So I launch a massive 'nice girl' campaign. The first week I befriend the porters. I confide in Charlie the blood porter and tell him how difficult it is for me to walk long distances. Soon he persuades all the porters to help me out. If I need anything taken anywhere I ring Charlie and he sorts it. I initiate a chocolate biscuit offensive with the nurses and secretaries and soon they are helping me out with routine tasks. I train my three best medical students to help with the bloods and I chat up the ward clerk. Before long everybody in the hospital knows me and I get the feeling they are all behind me. Soon the ward is running smoothly, leaving me time to deal with the more urgent medical problems. Each day I go home shattered and life at home is reduced to essential tasks only. Our tidy, friendly terraced house in West Derby village, Liverpool, looks as if it has been hit by a bomb.

Every third night I am on call, covering the acute surgical wards. Often I am up all night on my feet. Then I also have to work the following day. Sometimes I need to wear Lee-Roy III for stretches of 36 hours and at weekends I sometimes wear my leg non-stop for four whole days. The first time I have to do this I am in agony and my Little

Leg is chafed and sore. My phantom pains start up again, as they always do when I am tired.

But patients often give me something to keep me going. There is so much appreciation for what I am doing that somehow I manage it. I think of it as climbing a mountain. I just put one foot in front of the other. I have to get up to the top and come back down again without hurting myself too badly. By the end of the first week, though, my joints are swollen, my back aches and my Little Leg is covered with bruises.

Towards the end of it a new patient is admitted. I can see he is extremely unwell. He is very thin, pale and gaunt. I guess he must be thirty-something. His skin is sallow and waxy. His wife tells me he has been vomiting and has lost his appetite. When I examine his abdomen my hand encounters a hard, craggy lump. I feel for his liver – it is stony hard and bigger than it should be. I find lumps under his arms, too. He smiles at me, oblivious, and my heart sinks. The Limpet has struck another life. This time, though, it has advanced silently in a fatal ambush. The offspring of the Limpet are everywhere, silently sucking out his life.

'He has lost so much weight, too, Doctor. Is he going to be all right? He is all I have – we don't have any children yet, you see.'

'We need to run some tests,' I say, 'to find out what is wrong. Then I can tell you more.' I walk away with a heavy heart.

'Stomach cancer,' says Mr Cooke. 'Pretty advanced, I think. But we will take a look. List him for surgery, Mary.'

The operation is carried out next day. There is a huge, advanced cancerous growth. It is inoperable. The young man is going to die from his cancer. It is my job to tell him. I summon up every ounce of courage and compassion I can muster. We weren't taught how to do this at medical school. It isn't in the books. How do I tell a man in his early thirties he is dying?

I think back to the day Mr Peach told me about the cancer. What was it he said? 'You must be brave.' He held my hand and I knew he cared. He used the word 'cancer' so I could understand. He used the word 'death' so I knew the truth. I sit down with the young man and his wife. I hold his hand. For the first time I tell a patient he is facing death. The patient, his wife and I all cry.

'I am frightened,' he says.

'I know,' I reply. Because I do.

'Why me?' he asks.

'I don't know. I just don't know.' Because I don't.

'Thank you, Doctor. For being honest.'

'I'm so sorry.'

We sit in silence, listening to another Limpet advance.

I am so busy, the weeks pass very quickly. I am tired – exhausted – but I love being a doctor. I learn to deal with emergencies. I learn to talk to dying patients. I have never felt as content and valued as I do now.

Three months into my house job I face the inevitable. I knew it would happen one day.

'Mary,' says Mr Cooke at the end of the ward round, 'can I have a word?'

Mr Cooke is a fantastic consultant to work for. He is caring, humorous and dedicated. He expects me to work hard, knows I do not want any allowances made for me. In return he is one hundred per cent supportive.

'There is a patient coming in today. He has an osteosarcoma of his shoulder. We need to amputate his arm – a full forequarter amputation including his shoulder and collarbone.'

I draw my breath in sharply and look away.

'Are you going to be okay looking after him?'

'I guess so. I knew I would have to face it some time …'

'Yes, you do. Want me to see you through it?'

'Okay. I think I'm ready for it.'

'Do you think you're ready to assist me at the amputation in the operating theatre?'

'I'll try my best.'

Next day we meet in the scrub room.

'Let me know if you want out. No-one will think you can't cope. This is a difficult thing for you to face.'

I am glad a surgical mask is hiding my pale face. I stand opposite Mr Cooke in my green sterile gown and don my operating gloves. It feels a little like the day when I started my dissection – another hurdle to clear. This is the biggest I have yet faced.

'Ready, Mary?'

'Yes, ready.'

He hands me a large gauze swab and begins to cut. He explains everything he is doing and I concentrate on his voice. It is hot under the operating lights and I perspire. I can feel the droplets running down my nose.

127

'Okay, Mary?'

'Yes, I'm doing fine.'

I watch him carefully dividing the muscles that retain the arm in the shoulder joint. I feel very scared as the operation progresses. I cannot believe this was done to my body. The operation is brutal – radical and bloody. Soon the muscles are divided and Mr Cooke fashions the flaps of skin which will cover the wound and form the stump. My eyes fill up as he makes the final divisions and ties off the blood vessels. I blink the tears away quickly.

'Mary, I'm going to take the arm away now.'

In an instant, I think back to the day when I took the leg away from the cadaver in the dissection room. I remember how heavy it was. I feel terror as Mr Cooke lifts the arm with its shoulder attached and hands it to the waiting nurse. My hand brushes against the skin and I feel it, still warm with life. My mind escapes from my body as the severed arm falls with a heavy thud into the yellow bag. Mr Cooke has already captured the Limpet and trapped it in a pathology bucket. I look at the gore that remains of the exposed shoulder. The man's body is destroyed and mutilated. Looking at him now, I wonder if he will ever recover from the loss or escape the Limpet's further attack.

'Mary?' Mr Cooke brings me back to the stuffy operating room. 'You're one plucky woman,' he says.

There is relief as the nurse removes the yellow bag from the operating theatre. I wonder whether the patient remembered to say his farewells to his arm. I will ask him and, if he didn't, I can tell him I said goodbye for him instead.

'Ashes to ashes,' I think. 'Dust to dust.'

'Concentrate please, Mary,' says Mr Cooke. 'We need to close up the wound now.'

Blushing, I put my swab back in place.

After that, the remainder of my house year is never quite so difficult. I become used to the long hours and living in a sleepy twilight state. I build up my defences to cope with the emotional onslaught. I deal with every possible type of emergency and get used to the hectic pace of the hospital wards. The months pass and I become blunted to the pain and suffering all around me. There is no time to think deeply about what I encounter. I am merely numb with fatigue. It is a matter of survival. The faces and stories of my patients merge into a continuous blur of work to be done. I trudge through the work mechanically, exhausted but happy.

As July approaches my mind turns to my forthcoming wedding. I count down the days. The plans are just about finalized. The date is 15 July. The invitations have gone out. My designer wedding gown is hung carefully in the wardrobe. Everything is set to go. The last few weeks of my house job pass. Life seems to slow down as I wait for my wedding day to arrive but, finally, I am saying farewell to my colleagues, most of whom will be at the wedding.

'Bye bye, Dr Clewlow,' teases one of the patients. 'See you when you're Dr Self.'

I leave the ward with my heart singing. I have never felt so relieved to be walking out of the hospital as on this day. I make my way over to the doctors' residence, hand in my house officer's bleeper and throw my white coat into the laundry room.

'Bye bye, house year!' I rejoice, 'and good riddance, bleeper.'

I have made it through the year. I feel a gloating sense of achievement – there were several sceptics who advised me against attempting it full-time. Now it is complete and my job will never be as arduous again. In August I will take up a post as a senior house officer in anaesthetics at this same hospital, combining my love of acute medicine and the operating theatre. But first I have a wedding to attend!

The morning is a flurry of activity. Franny, Hellie and Sara cram into one room and put on their bridesmaids' dresses. They wear sky blue satin. Then my sisters and my mum help me prepare. They all stand back and admire my wedding gown. It is made of layer on layer of the softest cream silk with a beaded brocade bodice. They lift my cream veil over my face and fix it with a head-dress of fresh roses.

'Beautiful,' sighs my mum with tears in her eyes as she hands me my bouquet of heavily scented flowers.

I make my way downstairs and my dad looks at me proudly. As we climb into the vintage Rolls-Royce he turns to look at me. 'I never thought I would be doing this,' he says.

'Oh thanks a lot!' I joke. 'Did you think I'd end up on the shelf, then?'

'No. I honestly thought you would end up in a coffin.'

Suddenly I see how fragile my life is and has been.

'You look beautiful,' says my dad, then adds: 'Do you remember the ball gown your mum bought you?'

I wore it to the first medical ball I attended, shortly after my first cancer-free anniversary. My lilac silk dress was the envy of the entire year.

'I remember seeing it in the window,' I tell my dad as we drive towards the cathedral. 'I fell in love with it straight away – then saw the price label and walked away. When I turned round Mum was in the shop buying it for me!'

'Well, your mum didn't think she would ever be taking you to buy your wedding gown. That's why it meant so much to her to buy you that dress.' He takes my hands and adds: 'We are so proud of you and so happy you have found a loving man.'

I stand at the back of the cathedral chapel with my two sisters and Sara. It is packed with friends and colleagues. Many figures from my life are there – Mr Peach, John Jackett, my headmaster, Joan and Rita from medical school. I walk down the aisle to the sound of my brother Adrian playing on the organ the wedding march he has composed for us. I see Richard turn and smile at me. He watches as I reach the altar and prepares to lift back my veil. The wedding Mass begins and I recall the thought that popped into my head all those years ago, not a hundred yards from where we are now standing, that Richard had been chosen for me. I suppress a gleeful giggle as I marvel at the turns life takes. We exchange our vows and then say a special prayer we have written together.

'We pray that you will bless our home together with children,' I say.

'And that we will bring them up to love and serve the Lord,' continues Richard.

I add in my mind: 'Please answer this prayer. I cannot imagine a marriage without children. Please, God.'

Soon we are walking back down the aisle as man and wife and out into the glorious summer sunshine. I cast my eyes over the road to Ashton Street, where we first met.

'May I carry your skeleton, Dr Self?' Richard asks and, picking me up in his arms, he carries me down the cathedral steps ...

I am about to leave the casualty department but I am called back to see another patient. I have just completed a week of night shifts. Almost three years have passed since my marriage and I am now working as a casualty officer at the Royal Preston Hospital. I sigh as I read the details. Another elderly patient with chest pain. After I have taken a case history and completed my examination, a nurse helps me fill out the investigation forms.

'You look shattered,' she says.

130

'Just done a week of nights. It's been very busy.'

'Well, you can finish this one and then head off home to enjoy your days off. Who's on for medical emergencies?' She looks at the on-call list. 'Oh, it's Dr Self … are you related?'

'Yes, we're married.'

'Oh dear. He's on call all weekend. So you won't see him at all on your days off.'

'Nope,' I say curtly.

'Gosh – two doctors working full-time! When do you get to spend time together?'

'We don't. In fact, I'll probably call him to refer this lady and then I won't speak to him until Monday evening. Then I am on an evening shift, due in here again at 8.00 p.m. on Monday. He is on call again on Tuesday. Our next night together is Wednesday.' Seeing her quizzical look, I add: 'I suppose that's what it's like if you want to be successful in medicine. You have to put the hours in.'

Slowly I sigh and make the phone call to my husband who is working on a general medical ward at the same hospital.

'Hi, Richard. I'm really sorry but I've got a medical patient for you.'

'You're joking, aren't you?'

'No, I'm not – chest pain. I've done all the tests.'

'I've already taken three admissions this morning and it's only half past nine.'

'I know, it's this flu bug. They're coming in thick and fast.'

'Looks like I'm going to be a busy weekend. How was your night?'

'Awful.'

'When will I see you again?'

'Possibly Monday for half an hour – then Wednesday is our night off.'

'I'll probably be sleeping,' he says.

I sigh again and my heart sinks. 'Great,' I say.

'I can't help it. This job is a nightmare.'

'Is there any food in the house?'

'No, the freezer is empty.'

'Fantastic. I finish a week of nights and then have to shop too.'

'Look, I'm sorry, but I just crashed out last night, I was so shattered.'

'Don't you think I get shattered too?'

'I know you do. We are both overworked.'

'We need a holiday.'

'I can't take any for two months. There are too many juniors off – exam leave.'

'Richard, what are we going to do? Everything is going wrong. We just don't get time to talk or relax or anything. I am so worried about us.'

'I know. I feel the same way. It's like we have to book holiday to see each other.'

'We need to talk. I can't live like this any more.'

'Yes, we need to talk – it's just finding the time.'

'For goodness sake, we're married!' I am angry now and I lose my temper.

'Look, I haven't got time for this – I've got dozens of patients to see.'

'Fine!' I yell and slam down the phone, storming out of the casualty department in tears. The nurses watch me silently as I gather my stuff together and I know Richard and I will be their source of gossip for today.

I arrive back at our hospital flat and look around in dismay. The washing isn't done and there are pots and pans everywhere. There are at least two red bills to pay. I go to the fridge to make a cup of tea only to find we have run out of milk.

'*No*! I do not believe this!' I yell at the top of my voice. And I collapse on the bed in tears.

Throughout our marriage we have both worked full-time. We have both sailed through our post-graduate exams in anaesthesia and now we are taking time out to gain experience in other hospital specialities. But in the last six months our lives have fallen apart under the strain. Just lately it feels as if our marriage has been doing the same. We have argued badly.

The problem is lack of time. We are like ships passing in the night. We end up not talking and then little niggles become major arguments. Last week we talked about splitting up and I just don't know how we have got to this point. I look at our wedding picture beside the bed and wonder what is to blame.

'If I had children then I wouldn't have to put my career first,' I confide to my mum a little later. 'But that isn't going to happen. I feel like I have to give up either medicine or my marriage.'

'Can't you think of going part-time, darling?' she asks.

'I'd stuff my career.'

'Surely people would make allowances because of your disability?'

'But that's the whole point, Mum. I don't want to give in to my disability. If I do, then I feel as if the Limpet has won.'

132

I collect the mail and walk across the car-park with a heavy heart. How can we have lost the joy of our marriage and our medical careers? I used to love going to work and then I couldn't wait to come home. Now I don't look forward to either. I feel a sinking depression overwhelm me and decide I might as well pray. I haven't prayed properly for years now – not since I started medicine. There just hasn't been enough time. Something had to go, and it was my spiritual life.

'God, I don't know whether You are there,' I pray out loud. 'I don't even know if You care about me. But if You are there and if You do care, I need a sign. I know that it's not right to ask for signs because I'm meant to have faith. Sorry, God, I don't have any faith and I still need a sign. This is Your last chance. Do something – or I'm finished with You!'

The *British Medical Journal* is still in our pigeonhole from last week. I take it out and flick idly through the jobs section. My eyes are drawn to a large colourful advert for doctors in Australia.

It pictures a coral island under a blue sky. 'Come and work in sunny Queensland – good rates of pay – sociable hours – beautiful surroundings.' There is a tear-off slip to send for details.

'Why not? There's no harm in finding out,' I think to myself.

Towards the end of the week I arrive home to find Richard poring over a glossy brochure. 'Where did this come from?'

'I sent off for it. It was just one of those spur-of-the-moment things. I know it was a stupid idea.'

'No, Mary! It's not stupid. Have you seen this?' He hands me the brochure. There are scenes of the Great Barrier Reef and lush rain forest.

'It certainly looks beautiful, but there must be a catch.'

'I can't find one. There are some seminars to find out more. One's coming up next week. Shall we go?'

'It would be the answer to everything. We could gain more experience without having to work such barbaric hours.'

'We could contact John Wakefield too – he's working out in Queensland.'

'We need an adventure!' We grin at each other, suddenly united again in an exotic dream.

The following week, Richard heads off to the seminar without me because I have to work an extra shift. I am finishing it when he arrives. I am surprised to see him as we rarely visit each other's departments. He hands me an envelope.

'Open it,' he laughs. I tear it open. Inside I find a map of Australia. I look more closely and see a little cross.

'Is that where you would like to go?' I ask.

'Mary, that's where we are going!'

'What?'

'In six weeks' time!'

'We are going where?'

'Bundaberg, Queensland. Where John works. The hospital needs someone straight away. So I said that we could go in six weeks.'

I stare at Richard, completely speechless.

'You said you wanted to go …'

'Yes! I do! It's just that I didn't expect it to be so easy! Or so soon.'

Next day we hand in our resignations. 'No going back now!' he says.

'I don't want to go back. I've never been so unhappy.'

We mark the countdown to our departure on our calendar. There is so much to organize. With a week to go we are almost ready. We have our passports, our visas and our medical registration and our suitcases are packed. We have said most of our goodbyes and tidied up our gloomy hospital flat. Then I awake one morning feeling very unwell. I am due to start an early shift.

'Richard, I don't think I can make it into work today. I feel really poorly.'

'What's the matter?'

'I'm not sure. I feel so tired all the time,' I pause for a moment. 'I feel sick, too. It's just the last few days. And yet I'm so hungry.'

Richard looks at me curiously. 'Mary, when was your last period?'

Time seems to stop as I realize it was some time ago. 'I can't really remember. Quite a while back. I assumed it was late because of stress.'

'Mary, I think you must be pregnant!' Richard is laughing now.

'But … I can't be. I mean, it's not possible. The doctors said … I can't.'

'Yes, and the doctors also said that you would probably die and you didn't.'

'But what shall we do? We're going to Australia next week!'

'Let's make sure first and then cross that bridge.'

In the longest four minutes of my life, I sit in the bathroom waiting for the test to develop.

'You read it,' I tell Richard. 'I couldn't bear it to be negative now.'

I close my eyes while he reads the result. 'Please God! Please!'

134

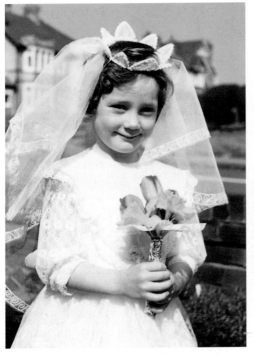

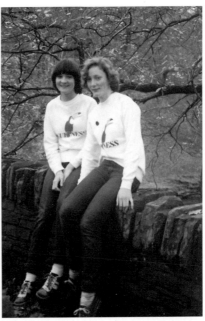

Mary and her sister Hellie on their Lake District walk, 1 November 1982, the day Mary made her Christian commitment.

Mary, aged seven, making her First Holy Communion.

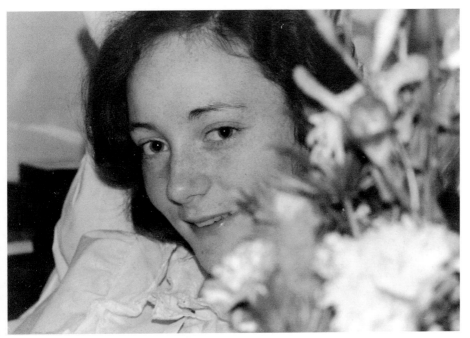

Mary, aged seventeen, three days after her amputation, in Ward 8, Victoria Hospital.

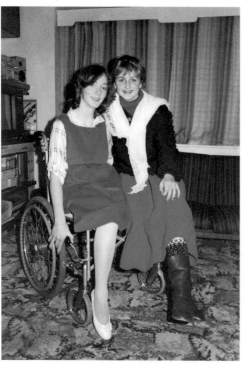

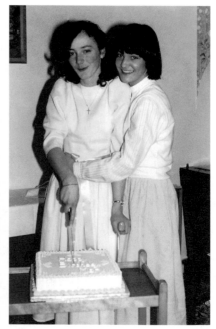

Mary and Hellie on 19 February 1983, celebrating Mary's eighteenth birthday.

Mary and her best school-friend, Adele, shortly after Mary's amputation in January 1983.

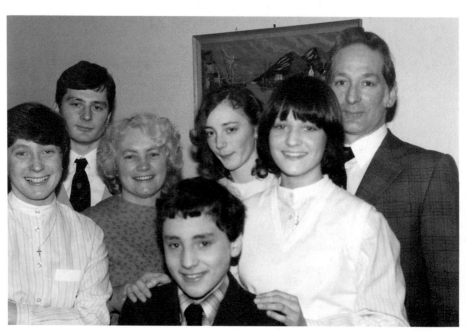

Mary and her family together on her eighteenth birthday weekend. (From left to right: Franny, Martin, Mum, Adrian, Mary, Hellie, Dad.)

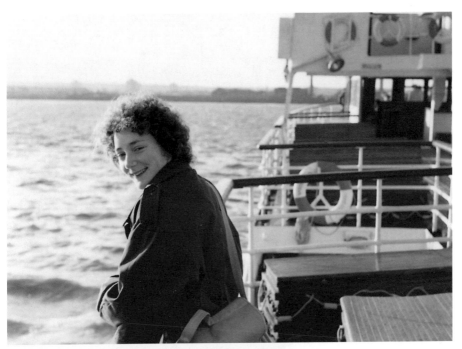

Mary on her first cancer-free anniversary, 7 January 1984, on the Mersey ferry where she would later become engaged.

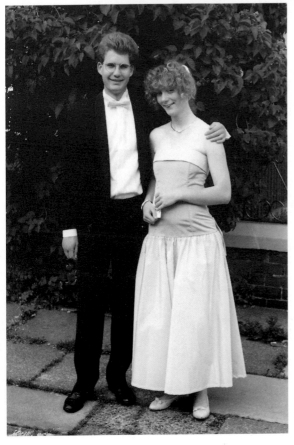

Mary and Richard at the Final Year Medical Graduation Ball in June 1988.

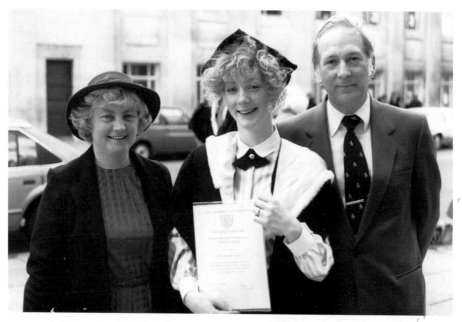

Graduating as Dr Mary Clewlow in June 1988 with her parents, Robert and Janet.

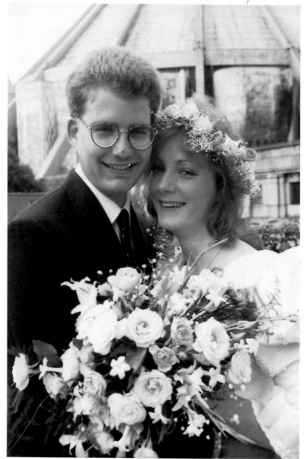

Mary and Richard on their wedding day, 15 July 1989, as she becomes Dr Mary Self.

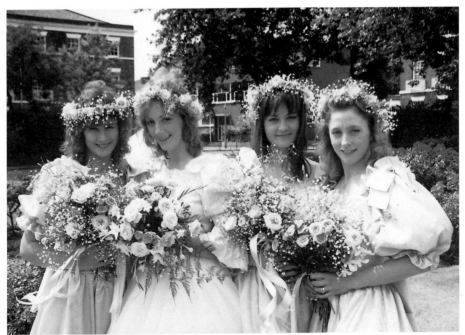

Mary with her bridesmaids:
fellow medic, Sara, and sisters,
Hellie and Franny.

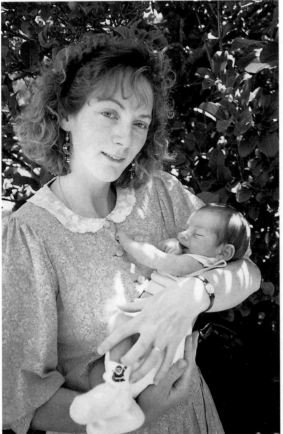

Mary with Adam, first
'miracle' baby on Christmas
Day 1992 in Australia.

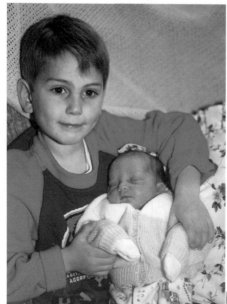

Adam, aged six, with newborn Bethany Lydia, second 'miracle' baby, 28 January 1998.

Mary with Adam, aged seven, and Bethany, aged one, in February 1999, shortly after her relapse was diagnosed.

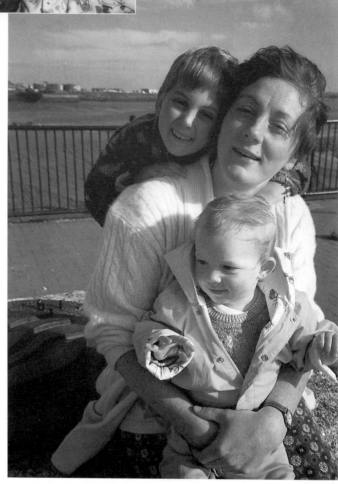

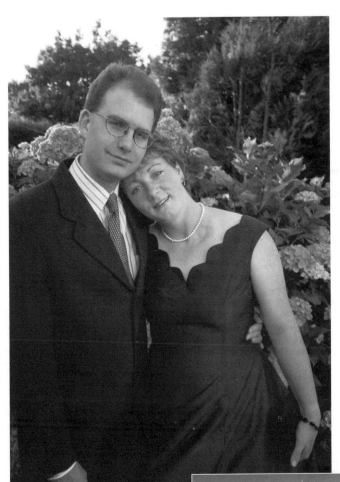

Mary – wearing the blue, sparkly dress she intended to be buried in – and Richard on their tenth wedding anniversary in July 1999, the last they anticipated sharing together.

Mary and Adam on Noosa beach, Queensland, August 1999, enjoying time on her 'final trip'.

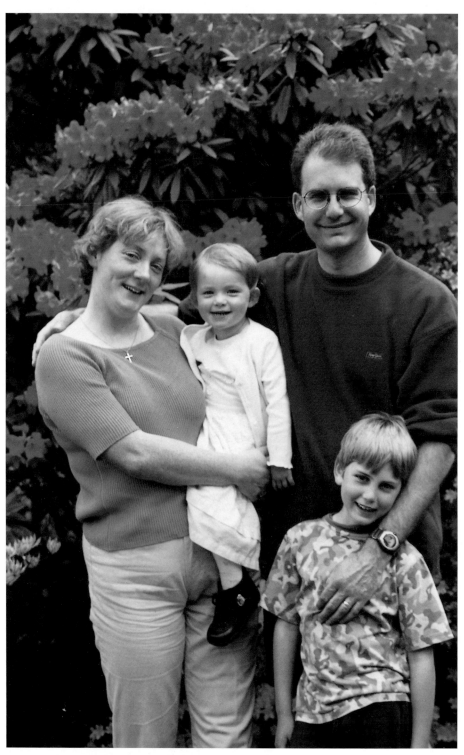

Mary with Richard, Adam and Bethany in May 2000, together as a family, six months after the third miracle.

'Mary – we're having a baby! You're pregnant!'

I cry loudly with indescribable joy. A baby! I thought it would never happen. God has answered the prayer!

'Mary. It's amazing.'

'What about Australia? Are we still going?'

'Do you want to?'

'Yes! Of course I do! A baby in Australia!' I remember asking God for a sign. I feel humbled as I remember how sceptical I was, and yet He still heard me.

I am eight weeks pregnant when we arrive in Queensland. It was a bit of a shock for our families when we told them we were having a baby and still travelling Down Under. But they were all soon excited at the prospect of an Australian child.

Stepping off the plane at Bundaberg airport is an unforgettable moment. It is April but the heat is incredible. The sky is completely clear and in the distance we can see palm trees swaying in the breeze. Our friend from medical school, John Wakefield, is there to meet us and show us round, helping us settle in. We discover that the first place we are going to be working in is a little town in the Outback called Eidsvold, a farming town with a high Aboriginal population. We will be the only doctors in a 50-mile radius, and a 5-hour drive from the nearest main hospital. It is a bit alarming to realize we will be responsible for the entire medical care of this community. From colds to post-mortems, we will be doing it all.

It feels like a real adventure as we are driven out back by the hospital driver. The scenery changes quickly from lush tropical coast to the dry and dusty roads of the interior. The baked red earth supports only stunted scrub and cacti. The horizon is dotted with kangaroos, emus and flocks of cockatoos streaked white against the dirt. Soon the cars are replaced by three-trailer road-trains, and even those become infrequent.

'So tell me what a couple of Poms are doing out back,' the driver asks.

'We got fed up of the hours back home,' we reply.

'And I hear the Rose is having a bub, too.'

'Pardon?'

'The lady – the English Rose. That's your pet name out here. Bub – that's baby. We heard you're expecting.'

'News travels fast, then.'

'Never faster. But listen now. You don't go driving out here on your own, you being pregnant. It's not safe.'

'Okay, I won't. But I'm fine, honest.'

'Listen. Out here, Rose, if you break down, you might not see another person for days. It's hot – you need water – and there are at least a dozen types of poisonous snake. One bite could see you under.'

'Sure – I'll be careful, I promise.'

'We don't want this baby hurt. We all feel responsible for you, Rose. It's two years since we had even one doctor out here. To get two is fantastic.'

This is our welcome to Eidsvold and it continues like that. We are made to feel like honoured guests for our entire stay. Within hours of arrival we have a car, a lovely air-conditioned home, a fridge full of food and dozens of invitations to supper. We become proud custodians of a twelve-bed hospital, an operating theatre and an X-ray machine. Our team includes ten nurses, two porters, an ambulanceman and a pilot! Soon we learn the joys and sorrows of every family in town. Outback life is tough but there is a loyalty and camaraderie unique to the great interior. People have learned to survive with very little and against the odds. I feel I belong.

My best friend in Eidsvold is an Aboriginal nurse. She is also called Vera.

'How's your momma feel 'bout you being out here?'

'Well, I guess a bit worried but then she has seen me come through a lot.'

'Yes, but your first child – it can be difficult to be on your own. I'm your momma while you're here, okay?'

Vera shares with me stories about the Aborigines and explains their way of life. She is full of helpful herbal remedies.

'I feel so sick!' I complain when morning sickness is at its worst.

'Raspberry leaf tea and I'll massage your wrists.'

There is a natural way to cope with everything. As my pregnancy progresses she calmly soothes the growing 'bub' when Baby becomes restless. 'Shh now – give your momma a break. Come on, tha's more like it …'

And it works. My somersaulting acrobat is soon peacefully sleeping.

Meanwhile, we deal with every imaginable medical situation. There are often times when we have to dredge our memories for medical student knowledge. But between us we seem able to cope. I look after obstetrics and casualty while Richard deals with paediatrics and medical. Major emergencies are stabilized and then transferred either by road to Bundaberg or by air to Brisbane. Not only do we diagnose and treat, but we also have to take all our own X-rays, apply our own plaster casts, administer anaesthetics and perform post-mortems if required. We meet some very unusual characters.

Every week we are asked to call at the local psychiatric residential home. On our first visit we pull up and are amazed to see a bright red London bus parked outside.

'Richard, I'm not hallucinating, am I?'

'It's definitely a London bus.'

We both look aghast at the rundown house. A verandah surrounds it and several rocking chairs creak eerily, occupied by bedraggled patients.

'I'm Kitty, I run the place.' A plump motherly figure greets us. 'Come on and meet all my friends.'

The patients are all schizophrenics on long-acting medication. We give the injections and then settle on the verandah with a glass of home-made lemonade.

'We were wondering about the bus, how it came to be here,' I ask Kitty.

'I drove it from Sydney. Don't know how it got to Sydney.'

'Why did you drive a bus from Sydney?'

'To bring this lot here. Most of them were homeless. I went round, asked them if they needed a home and we drove out here in the bus. Been here ever since. That was ten years ago. I guess when we get fed up we'll drive somewhere else.'

Kitty lifts an arm to wave to a man riding a bicycle. I glance at him and then have to look twice. He has a cockatoo chained to the handlebars.

'That's George and the cockatoo is Joey. He takes it everywhere. It's like a child to him.'

Richard and I look at each other: the Outback is full of eccentrics. In terms of both geography and normality, we are thousands of miles from home.

One blistering hot day we decide to picnic and head for the muddy creek which is the only water for miles. We have become used to beating the long grass with sticks to check for king brown snakes – one bite can prove instantly fatal. We watch the herons fishing and the troops of pink and grey galahs squawking noisily. Suddenly, in the distance, we see the ambulance driving towards us, the driver beckoning us to head back to the hospital. When we get back we find a herdsman who has been thrown from his horse.

'The horse rolled on him,' the nurse tells us. 'He dragged himself five miles to get here.'

We examine him. His pelvis is badly broken and beads of sweat stand out on his brow.

'We need to give you some painkillers,' I say to him.

'No, Doctor – I don't want any.'

I look at him. He is smiling – more grimacing – his pulse rate is very high and his blood pressure raised. Obviously he is in a great deal of pain.

'We can easily give you some morphine …'

'No, Doctor, I'd just as soon go without.'

I turn, bewildered, to the nurse, who signals me to leave. 'The herdsmen won't have painkillers. They think they need to be tough,' she explains. So our herdsman with a smashed pelvis smiles through his five-hour road trip to Bundaberg without the aid of morphine.

We deal with car accidents, snake bites and wasp stings. We immunize children, stitch wounds and fix fractures. We pack a tree-feller's severed hand in ice for re-implantation after staunching the haemorrhage – a chainsaw injury. We have two weekends off in three months but we have never been happier in our work. Something happens, too, as Richard and I work together as a team and share our knowledge and our workload. We fall in love with medicine again and we fall back in love with each other.

In July 1992, after three months in Eidsvold, we leave the tiny town and wave until our friends are out of sight.

'We will come back one day,' I say to Richard. 'When our child is big enough, we'll return and show him the Outback.'

'Yes, and it will probably all still look the same. The only thing that might have changed is the London bus, which might have moved on.'

We move back to Bundaberg, a larger coastal town at the southern tip of the Great Barrier Reef and on the aptly named Sunshine Coast. For the visitor, life in Bundaberg revolves around the beach and the sea. In July, winter temperatures are still warm and every single day brings blue skies. The hospital provides us with a flat and we spend our free time exploring the beautiful beaches. We make many close friends who become our substitute family. Chris and Janelle are our Aussie neighbours. They teach us about the Australian way of life. John Wakefield, his wife Angela and their little girl are living at the hospital, so we see a lot of them and they give us a great deal of help planning the birth of our baby. Another new friend, Tim, is a British social worker. He teaches me everything about relaxing on a beach! We are now all excitedly awaiting my baby's arrival. The atmosphere at the hospital is happy and relaxed and there are plenty of other British doctors out here.

My bump becomes too big for me to walk easily and I am offered a hospital job working in the psychiatric unit. I haven't worked in this area of medicine before. I am not expecting to enjoy it but, surprisingly, I do. I find my experiences of grief and my moments of despair help me understand my patients in a way I had not imagined. It also means I can work without risking my mobility. My artificial leg is not meant to carry this amount of weight and I am very slow and ungainly. I get a lot of phantom pain, too, where Baby presses on the nerves in my pelvis. The belt around what used to be my waist is very uncomfortable and I don't think Baby likes it much, either, because I get kicked furiously whenever I walk!

Even so, I feel very fortunate to know that, at last, after all my hopes and prayers, the time is drawing near when I will hold my own baby. Everything seems to be going well. The pregnancy has been trouble-free and the ultrasound scans seem to show my baby has not been harmed by the chemotherapy I received ten years ago; it would be typical of the Limpet to launch a counter-attack.

I have enjoyed every moment of my pregnancy. I love to watch the baby I thought I would never have growing bigger. I love to feel the tiny kicks under my ribs. Sometimes I just lie and talk to Baby and think how wonderful it is that the doctors were wrong after all.

In my last month of pregnancy, Richard returns from a dive trip full of the wonders of the reef. I feel a little envious because I have not been able to dive or snorkel for fear of harming Baby.

'The coral was amazing!' he tells me. 'I saw brightly coloured angel fish and huge flapping manta rays. We even saw sharks and sea snakes!'

'I'm so glad you had a great time,' I reply, 'but I'm even happier you're back. Now I don't have to worry about giving birth alone!'

Twenty-four hours later we are watching a film when I feel a huge gush of warm fluid soak my chair. An excruciating pain takes my breath away.

'Richard – help! The baby is coming!'

My contractions come thick and fast and soon I am gasping with pain. 'Oh, God, I never thought it would be like this. Take it away, please!'

Richard drives the mile across town to the maternity unit in record time. 'It's okay, we're here now,' he reassures me as he drags me through the door of the labour ward. Soon I am settled in a delivery room and the journey I have watched so many times becomes reality for me.

'Push! Come on! You're nearly there!' the midwife urges.

'I can't!'

'You can!' Richard and the midwife yell in unison.

'It hurts, oh God, it hurts!'

I never thought I would see this day and the pain, though terrible, is also exquisite and infinitely pleasurable. It merges with victory as I push my baby out into the world and look upon my perfect, healthy son.

'A boy! It's a boy!' says Richard. 'What shall we call him?'

'Adam – of the red clay. First-fruit. Australian child.'

'Welcome to the world, Adam!'

Richard kisses his son proudly and gently, his lips resting on the soft wet skin.

Ten years ago I prayed for three miracles.
Ten years on, an unlooked-for miracle.
Adam, my son. Thank you, God.

9

It is May 1993. We have returned home to the UK and introduced our Australian child to our families, settling and obtaining junior doctor posts in South Wales. It is an area of the country with which neither Richard nor I have previous connections. But, after a year spent living next to an Australian beach, we need to be near the sea. We choose Swansea, which has easy access to the Gower and Pembrokeshire coasts. Richard and I both continue to work in the field of anaesthetics, at Morriston and Singleton hospitals. I manage to organize a part-time post, enabling me to enjoy motherhood, too.

On 7 January 1993, before leaving Australia, we marked my tenth cancer-free anniversary. I celebrated in style, also welcoming baby Adam – a month old to the day – and saying goodbye to our Australian friends. The group of which we had become a close part was breaking up and we were going our separate ways. Richard and I were moving back to the United Kingdom. A month with a colicky baby convinced me I needed my mum around! Following a rowdy barbecue and lots of champagne I lay on the beach beside our friend Tim. He had been our chief baby-sitter and main support during the chaotic four weeks since Adam's birth. The night was hot and humid and Adam lay peacefully asleep, at last, on a blanket beside us.

'So, how does it feel to be ten years down the line from your cancer?'

'Fantastic – and even better because of Adam being here. Babies weren't supposed to be possible. To survive ten years, yes, this is significant.'

'Are you cured?'

'As cured as I ever will be. This type of cancer relapses early, so ten years is a major milestone. It's the goal I always set myself, to be discharged from medical care.'

'Well, here's to a cure and a beautiful baby too! Cheers!'

By the time we have settled into our new jobs and new home, Adam is a busy and cheerful baby of eight months. The only unfulfilled aspect of my life is my faith. After Adam was born I needed to find a way back to God. I guess in those precious moments following the birth, when I looked upon my son with so much joy, I realized He had not abandoned me.

One fine autumn day I am playing with Adam in the garden when a neighbour stops to chat.

'Hello, I'm Jean. I live up the other end of the road.'

'Oh, hello. We've just moved in. I'm Mary and this is Adam.'

'Well, I'm just off to help with the mother and toddler group at the church hall. I was wondering if you wanted to come?'

'I'm not too sure – it isn't really my thing …'

'Nonsense!' Jean says briskly. 'You need to meet other mums and Adam needs to make friends. I know you'll enjoy it.'

'Parklands Evangelical Church …' I read from the sign. The building looks like a rather run-down community hall. Inside, dozens of toddlers are running around crazily. A helper comes over to me, smiling warmly.

'Hello, I'm Alison. I run the group and also help out at the church. Come and sit down and tell me about yourself.'

I can't help but warm to the kindness and friendship. I go regularly to the Monday group. All the helpers are members of the church. As Christmas 1993 approaches a party is planned – Adam's first Christmas party. I look forward to it excitedly. On the day, however, he awakes grumpy, unwell and covered in a rash from head to foot. Soon he is refusing feeds and vomiting. The day passes in a depressing whirl of changing nappies and bedclothes; thoughts of the party are forgotten. Eventually, in the late afternoon, an exhausted Adam finally sleeps and I sit down to rest. I am dirty and tired and completely disorganized. Richard is on call at the hospital overnight and I feel lonely and worried. As I doze in the chair, I hear a knock at the door.

'Is everything all right, Mary? We missed you at the party.'

Tearfully I explain my predicament of a sick child, no Calpol, a house full of wet washing and nothing for tea.

'Don't worry,' Alison reassures me. She leaves with bags full of cot sheets. She returns loaded with piles of freshly tumbled linen, a casserole and a large bottle of Calpol.

'Now if you need anything in the night, just ring us.' She hands me a Parklands Church pamphlet and explains that her husband, Brian, is an Elder.

Closing the door, I think maybe I will attend a service just to see what it's like.

On the first Sunday of 1994 I make my way to church. The anniversary of my operation is approaching and making me rather contemplative. The night is dark and cold and the rain is teeming. I hug my coat as the wind whips around me, causing me to shiver. But, walking across the church car-park, I hear the loud noise of joyful singing. As I arrive, a tall, bearded man shakes my hand, saying: 'It's so lovely to see you here with us tonight.' I push the door and walk in. The hall is bare save for a wooden cross on the wall and some colourful banners with scripture verses. It is packed with people of all ages. Happiness shines from their faces. I notice one of my 'mother and toddler' friends and she waves. The words of the hymn are displayed on an overhead screen. The tune is unfamiliar, and I feel hesitant and uncertain, but I stand at the back and read the words:

> Father God I wonder
> how I managed to exist
> without the knowledge of your parenthood
> and your loving care.
> But now I am your child
> I am adopted in your family
> and I will never be alone
> for Father God
> you're there beside me …

Suddenly a wall of sensation hits me. It is like a surge of physical power. It is as if a huge pair of arms is grabbing hold of me, shaking me back to reality. My whole body feels stronger, straighter and I am filled with amazing peace and joy as, for the first time since the night before my operation, I hear the voice of the Presence again speaking into my mind. Through a sound like a powerful waterfall I can make out the words: 'You're back.'

I cry real salty tears as I become aware of my faith returning – faith as I knew it all those years ago when I awoke in my hospital bed on Ward Eight and first met the Presence. In an instant I see clearly that the seed of my faith has lain dormant and struggled to grow through all the dark days of my illness. I have tried and tried to make it grow but it has never been watered and so the leaves have never sprouted. There were moments when I glimpsed a few drops of rain, but the pain and despair of the Limpet were too great for me. A supernatural hand beyond my understanding has brought me through the years of drought somehow. Now, it is as if I am standing under the huge waterfall I can hear in my head, drinking in the goodness of all that I have missed out on. It is as if the desert of my soul, soaked by the downpour, has burst forth into wonderful and exotic bloom.

'Yes! I'm back. I am really back!'

This is the most significant day of my spiritual life since the Limpet – the day that I come back to knowing God for real. At Parklands Evangelical Church I grow up in my Christian faith. I learn the importance of praying regularly and not just when I feel like it. By attending church every week and going to teaching events I begin really to understand the scriptures. Soon the Bible I had previously read only superficially becomes familiar at a much deeper level and I hunger daily to read it. One day I share the story of the Presence with Brian and Alison, who have become my spiritual mentors.

'I've always wondered about the Presence. Who was it? Was it real or was I out of my mind on drugs?'

'No, I think what you describe is a real and true physical presence of God; maybe an angel, maybe the Spirit of God,' Brian explains, as if it is something that happens all the time.

'An angel? I thought they had haloes, dressed in tinsel and sang "Silent Night"!'

Brian laughs. 'No, there are quite a lot of reports of experiences like yours – especially at times of extreme trauma, near-death events and severe illness. We can never know for certain, but it was obviously some very powerful encounter with God, possibly to prepare for what you then had to go through.'

As I grow in faith and knowledge, my life begins to change in other ways. I worry less and become more patient. Situations which once would have caused me anxiety and fear seem manageable. The difficulties of living with a disability become easier. My frustration with my limitations lessens and I grow in self-confidence. But, as 1995 dawns and our family and working lives become busier, I find the physical strain of my job in anaesthetics too great. I make the decision to retrain in the field of psychiatry, allowing me more time and energy to devote to my family.

In the summer of 1995 we come to the end of our stay in Swansea. Richard is due to start work in the University Hospital of Wales in Cardiff, progressing in his anaesthetics career. My post in psychiatry is to be based in Cardiff, at the Whitchurch Hospital. Throughout our time in Swansea, Richard has been very impressed by the love Parklands Evangelical Church has shown us. He has attended churches sporadically during the twelve years we have been together but he has never made his own personal profession of faith. The day before we leave Swansea, surrounded by the friends who helped me to rediscover my own faith, Richard's Christian faith is born. We move to Cardiff and attend the evangelical Rhiwbina Baptist Church.

The following year, 1996, passes peacefully and life is calm and settled. Adam grows into a happy and contented little schoolboy, full of fun and mischief. Richard and I both settle into our new jobs and, as a family, we share far more time together as a result of my change in medical disciplines. Our church family at Rhiwbina Baptist is both loving and supportive, and we all grow stronger in our faith.

As my fourteenth anniversary arrives in 1997, we have some great news to celebrate. We are expecting our second child.

'Richard – the test is positive!' I call from the bathroom. I remember the Romany Christian's prophecy. 'It will be a girl – I know! I just know it!'

'So have you thought of a name for Baby?'

'Yes, she's going to be called Lydia Mary. I must be a long way on in the pregnancy. It's a couple of months since I had my period and the test is very strongly positive. I've worked it out as fifteen weeks.'

The following day I feel Lydia move. The familiar little flutters make me squeal with delight.

'Richard, I just felt the baby move!'

'When will my sister be born, Mummy?'

'Sometime in the summer, darling. It takes a long time to grow a baby.'

'When will we know if it really is a girl?'

'When Mummy has a scan – it's like seeing it on television.'

Adam seems as excited as we are about the new baby.

January 16 begins like any other day. I have the usual couple of hours of morning sickness, dashing back and forth to the toilet. My scan is booked for next week and I am really looking forward to seeing Lydia for the first time. My pregnancy is just beginning to show and

145

I have already done some baby shopping. I drag myself home after a busy day at work and rest on the bed, determined to do everything possible to keep the pregnancy healthy. I have been following all the advice and the midwife is very pleased with my general state of health.

Suddenly I become aware of a sharp pain spreading across my lower back. I sit up and see a pool of blood spreading across the bedclothes.

'Richard, come here quickly,' I shout. 'Something is happening. Oh no! Richard, help – I'm losing Lydia!'

'Lie down quickly.' Richard rushes in. 'I'll call the doctor.' I lie on my side, petrified. The life-blood of my daughter is seeping away and there is nothing I can do to stop it. I pray over and over again: 'Please don't let her die. Don't let her die. She is already part of my life. Don't take her away from me. She is meant to be born. The prophecy told me!'

By the time the doctor arrives the bleeding has stopped, but he insists on me going to hospital straight away and phones for an ambulance. Soon Richard and I are in a side ward awaiting the arrival of the specialist.

'Nigel Davies is the consultant on call tonight,' Richard reassures me. 'He's the best gynaecologist in the hospital. He will look after you. I talked to him just now and he is coming in to see you.'

I don't have long to wait before there is a knock on the door.

'Hi, I'm Nigel, and I'm very sorry to hear that you're not well.' He smiles in a kindly fashion and sits on the edge of the bed, asking me the usual questions about the pregnancy and my dates.

'I'm sixteen weeks. I thought by now everything would be going well. I didn't think this could happen so late.'

'Well, you might have got your dates muddled,' he suggests, 'but let's take a look and see.' He smiles at me as he prepares the ultrasound scan to look at the baby.

'I'm going to be looking for the baby's heart,' he explains. 'We should be able to see it clearly by now. Do you want me to tell you what I am seeing?'

'Yes, I do. Please tell me the truth. I need to know.'

He positions the ultrasound screen so I cannot see it. I know that is unusual and I feel scared – he must be expecting bad news. Then he searches around to find a clear picture of the womb.

'Okay, I've found your womb now and I can see the placenta. I'm going to measure it … fifteen weeks' size.'

146

'That's good then, is it?' I am desperate to hear that Lydia is unharmed, but there is a silence. Nigel is peering at the screen closely.

'Mary – it's not good news.'

'No,' I cry, 'don't tell me that.'

'I'm not getting a heartbeat. The baby is much smaller than your placenta ...'

'What does that mean?'

'Mary, I'm sorry. I can't find the heartbeat. Your baby is dead.'

'Dead? Is there really no hope?'

'No, Mary, none at all. I'm so sorry. I think your baby died a few weeks ago. That would account for it being smaller than the placenta.'

'But how – I mean, why? I did everything right.' I am crying, angry that my body has betrayed me. All those weeks I thought I was pregnant and Lydia was lying dead in my womb, a tiny little corpse in a placenta tomb.

'I think probably there was some major congenital problem for the baby to be so underdeveloped, but we can only know for sure by sending off the embryo for tests.'

Lydia has suddenly become less than a baby. In medical terms, she is now an embryo that my body will soon reject. All the hopes and plans I had made for my tiny child are over. I feel numb with shock and grief. I place a hand protectively over my womb. I am not ready to let go of her.

'Do you want me to take the placenta away, Mary ... and the baby?'

'Not yet. I don't know. I don't feel ready.'

'Okay.' Nigel nods understandingly. 'How about I give you some time to think? We can always do an operation first thing tomorrow.'

'Nigel, was it my fault? Was it anything I did?' I feel so guilty that I could not provide a life for my child. I feel a failure, almost as if my body has not passed the test.

'No, Mary. If the pregnancy wasn't healthy there was nothing you could have done to save it.'

'What about the chemotherapy?'

'What chemotherapy?'

'When I was younger. I mean, could that have affected it? I had high doses of Methotrexate for my bone cancer, and I had isotopes as well.'

'Well ... I suppose it's possible that some of your eggs were damaged, but we can't know for sure. You mustn't blame yourself; mostly we never know the reason.'

Nigel leaves the room with Richard and I hear them talking quietly outside. I have been aware of a baby within me and now I am alone again. My baby can no longer hear the steady beat of my heart; her own little heart has stopped. I turn and look out of the window into the dark night. I feel so empty. Then I feel the familiar surge of anger.

'Stupid thieving Limpet, it's all your fault,' I think. 'If you hadn't showed up, I would never have had chemotherapy, Lydia would still be here, my leg would still be here. You take everything away. You're an evil thieving murderer.'

It feels good to blame the Limpet again and make it into the villain once more. There will never be any punishment big enough for the damage it has caused in my life. There will never be any forgiveness now – not now it has caused my child to die, too. I lie in my bed that night and watch my baby's life-blood slowly spreading in a red pool on the starched white hospital sheets. With every new gush of warm stickiness I whisper in my mind: 'I hate you Limpet. I hate you.'

Over the next few weeks I live in a twilight world of sorrow. I awake every morning with thoughts of Lydia in my mind and reality hits me with the full force of a physical blow as I experience the loss all over again. 'Richard, she's gone, hasn't she?' And the black cloud descends for the rest of the day. It feels as if nothing will ever take it away. Hugs, gifts, flowers, even cuddles from Adam feel meaningless beside what I have lost. It is hard to understand how an unborn baby whom I have never seen could cause so much pain. And yet it is the not seeing that makes it so difficult. I have nothing to remind me of her – no teddy, no photograph … it is just a big black hole of misery.

My grief is not helped by a nagging awareness that my body is not completely well. Over the next few months I develop complications from the loss of my baby. One morning I awake to find myself haemorrhaging heavily again. I manage to crawl to the telephone and summon help from a friend before I collapse from the blood loss. Once more I need further surgery. Following this, I experience severe chronic pain in my pelvis but all the tests are unhelpful.

'I'm not sure what's going on, Mary,' Nigel tells me. 'I guess that you are just being a typical doctor – a problem from beginning to end.'

Deep down I begin to wonder if the symptoms are related to the Limpet. I push the thoughts firmly away, putting them down to my fragile mood. If I accept the thoughts then I will have to do something about them and all I can think about is becoming pregnant again. It seems as if, everywhere I go, happy and healthy babies abound. It becomes impossible to pass a baby or a pregnant woman without tears springing to my eyes. The urge to hold another child is so strong and yet, when I do, I sob so much that I have to hand it back. Even seeing baby clothes arouses in me a stream of black, depressing thoughts. As the weeks go by, everybody forgets Lydia apart from me. She will always be there, a part of my life. I see in my mind's eye how she would have looked in her sweet pink baby dresses and I can feel exactly how her little hands would have curled around my own.

Giving her an identity helps me let go of her. I buy a beautiful box and fill it with gifts I have been given by my friends in the weeks following her death. I put in the baby clothes I bought for her and some of the cards and dried flowers I received. One of my friends, Ruth, works as a bereavement counsellor and helps me arrange a memorial service. I feel I should say goodbye in some way. It reminds me of the day Richard, Judith and I gathered in the university chapel and said goodbye to my left leg. As I gather once again with my close friends and family, I realize grief comes in many different forms. We read scriptures and sing hymns before I seal up Lydia's box and say my final farewell to her. After this, although I never forget her, I am able to move on and think about the future again.

In May 1997 I discover I am pregnant again. The delight I have felt hitherto when discovering my pregnancies is this time replaced by an acute sense of fear. I was warned following the complications which arose after my haemorrhage that I was at risk of developing an ectopic pregnancy, so it becomes vital to make sure at an early stage that the baby is lying in the womb. I ring Nigel nervously and tell him my news.

'That's great, Mary! Congratulations!'

'You're not allowed to say that until the baby is born this time,' I say. 'I'm not getting my hopes up again. I'm only six weeks pregnant.'

'Well, let's scan you this week, then. How about Thursday, two days' time? If we see a heartbeat at six weeks then that is a very good sign.'

I await my scan impatiently. It feels as if it is going to be the longest two days of my life. On the Wednesday morning I wake early, feeling very nervous again. As I step into the shower I am hit by a wall of pain in my abdomen. I double up, gasping. I try to stand upright but I cannot. I began to feel excruciating pain in my shoulder tip – a diagnostic sign of a ruptured ectopic pregnancy and ruptured ectopics can be fatal.

'O God,' I whisper through clenched teeth, 'You have to do something.'

I am in so much pain, I cannot even take in a breath to scream. I am vaguely aware of Adam wandering into the bathroom.

'What are you doing on the floor, Mummy?'

'Get Daddy – now …' Adam begins to cry and runs off to fetch his dad.

'Daddy!' he shouts. 'Mummy is on the floor. I think the baby is dying again,' and I hear his loud howls. He went through his own sense of loss after Lydia died.

'God,' I pray as Richard comes into the bathroom. 'I don't think I can go through this again. I really don't.'

'Mary?' I can feel Richard taking my pulse. 'Mary, can you hear me?'

'It hurts – my belly. My shoulder, too …'

'Shit!' I hear Richard curse under his breath. 'Mary, I'm going to call an ambulance, okay? Just hold on.'

I feel dizzy and sick and everything goes round and round. The voices of Adam and Richard seem to go quiet and then loud again.

'God, save my baby, please.'

'What's wrong with Mummy? Why won't she answer you?'

'Mummy has a sore tummy. Go and look out for the ambulance.'

'I'm dying. Don't let me die.'

'Mary? Mary? Squeeze my hand. The ambulance is on its way.'

'Mummy, Mummy, Mummy – wake up!'

'She's up here. Looks like it's a ruptured ectopic. Her pulse is very weak.'

'Do you want to put a drip in?'

'I'll not get one in here. Her veins are dreadful. Scoop and run.'

They try to move me. 'No … no, it hurts.' My abdomen feels as if it is on fire.

'Breathe this,' and a mask is stuck over my face. It smells sweet and soon I am all floppy. Then I am in the back of an ambulance and everything is moving really fast. There are sirens and lights and I realize it is me being carried, not someone else.

'Mary, stay with us. We're almost at the hospital.'

And then I am rushed through the doors and there are bright lights and a man leaning over me, wearing a mask.

'Mary, I'm going to put a drip in. Keep still.'

I roll around in agony.

'Shall I give her some morphine, Doctor? She is in so much pain.'

'No, her pressure's too low. We need to give her some fluid and see what is going on first.'

Then I black out and, next thing I know, I am back in that horrible room where I had my scan last time I almost bled to death. Someone is shoving something up my vagina and I don't know what is happening to me. I try to get up and see but a nurse pushes me back.

'We need to see the baby.'

'It hurts! It hurts, get off me.'

'There's blood everywhere in the pelvis. She's bleeding from somewhere. About a litre.'

Oh God. How can a baby survive that?

'Hang on – what's that? It's a pregnancy, in the womb, look. There's a tiny heartbeat. But where's the blood coming from?'

I am struggling to get up again – 'It hurts, please stop the pain' – and I hear Richard's voice, 'Look, you've got to give her something, she is in agony,' and then I am hit by a whoomph of something like an intense orgasm and my pain disappears completely and instantly.

As I descend into unconsciousness I hear a voice saying, 'Your baby is still alive, Mary.'

'Thank you …' Then there is silence.

'Mary? Mary … are you awake?' I turn my head slowly and see Nigel's grey eyes peering into mine.

'What happened? Is my baby alive?'

'Your baby is alive and so are you. You've been sleeping off the morphine.' He puts his fingers on my pulse and I see I am receiving a fast-flowing intravenous drip of blood substitute.

'It's a good job Richard was at home with you.'

'I thought it was a ruptured ectopic.'

'So did everyone else!'

'So what caused all the pain?'

'You bled into your pelvis from an ovarian cyst. We need to scan you again to see whether the bleeding has stopped.'

'But the baby – you're sure the baby is alive?'

'The baby was alive when we did the scan before. We are going to take you down again just now. I'll come with you and the senior radiologist is going to have a look and see.'

'Will I be okay, Nigel? It was so scary. I thought I was going to die.'

'You almost did. You lost an awful lot of blood. You'll be okay now you are here.'

151

A little later the radiologist turns the scanner screen round for me to see. 'There we are – Baby is alive, you can see his heart.'

'Her heart. It's a girl. I know it's a girl.'

'Well, it's something of a miracle she made it after you lost so much blood, but she seems none the worse for her traumatic day. Look, she is even turning around for you,' and I see the baby wriggle in my womb.

'Tough baby,' jokes Nigel, 'just like her mother. From now on, Mary, I'll call you Heartsink.'

'Are you going to operate?' I ask.

'Well, it's your choice. If we remove the cyst surgically then we would have to take the ovary and you would lose the baby. If we treat you conservatively, with bedrest, then we run the risk of a re-bleed but it is your best chance of keeping the baby.'

'No, I've seen this baby now and I know what she has been through. If it turns out to be an ovarian cyst then I will take the risk of a re-bleed. I want to keep this baby.'

So I remain on bed-rest for the first third of my pregnancy and the problems settle down. Nigel scans the baby each week to keep a check on her and reassure me. Soon I feel I know my baby very well. As I reach the sixteenth week of pregnancy, I begin to relax a little. I know the chances of losing this baby are now much smaller. As my bump grows bigger I find it more and more difficult to get around. I found it difficult to walk during my first pregnancy but this time the problems are worse and, for some reason, I am experiencing pelvic pain most of the time. I guess it is due to the internal bleeding I had at the start of the pregnancy.

By the time I am eight months pregnant I have planned the arrival of our new baby completely. The cot is assembled, the nappies purchased and the shiny designer pram stacked in the corner of the garage. Adam is becoming more and more excited at the prospect of a baby sister. I am becoming more and more immobile and when, at 37 weeks, I am more or less totally housebound, Nigel becomes concerned.

'Mary, if you fall badly you could injure yourself and the baby. I think we should go for an induction of labour.'

'I am finding it really difficult, to be honest. I can't even take Adam to school at present because the hill is too steep for me to walk up.'

'Okay, then – come into the ward on Monday with your bags packed!'

The following Monday we drop Adam at school and head for the University Hospital.

'It seems strange knowing that in a few hours we will have our baby with us,' I say as I climb on to the bed. 'I'm sure that it won't take long second time around …'

'Richard, I can't take any more of this pain,' I weep the following day. 'I've been in labour since yesterday. It's lunchtime now, and I'm so tired. I feel like giving up.'

'Come on, you're nearly there now. It won't be much longer.'

I scream in agony as another furious contraction takes over. 'Oh please, let this baby be born soon!'

A few hours later, after a long and exhausting labour, my baby decides to make an entrance.

'About time too!' jokes the midwife as she delivers the baby's head. 'And now for the moment of truth …' She gently pulls my second child out into the world and places the slimy, wriggly bundle on my tummy.

'It's a girl!' she laughs. 'What are you going to call her?'

I am laughing and crying with relief and joy. 'My darling, darling, daughter. I waited so long for you! I never thought I would hold you!' I cry as I hold her to my breast. 'Bethany. You are called Bethany Lydia.'

Bethany – the place where Jesus called forth His dead friend Lazarus from the tomb and made him live again.

Bethany Lydia – miracle daughter.
The second miracle.
Thank you, God.

10

I have never really picked up since giving birth to Bethany.

She grows from strength to strength, but it seems as if my own life is being drained. As she smiles and chuckles, I feel gloomy and sad. I look at my daughter and love her so much. She is a constant source of joy and sunshine but I can sense a shadow creeping over me. My thoughts return time and again to the Limpet. I experience the same unsettling fear I lived with so long ago. The physical pain I have experienced since the death of Lydia continues and becomes worse. I become used to living with a constant nagging ache in my left side. Eventually I pluck up courage and return to hospital. I arrange to see Nigel in clinic and tell him my fears.

'I can't help wondering if it's something to do with the bone tumour. It's too late for a secondary, but maybe I've developed another type of cancer.'

'Well, it's very unlikely after all these years.'

'I know and I realize I'm probably just worrying. But maybe I've got cancer somewhere else; in my ovary, perhaps.'

'Let's have a look, then. Hop on the couch and I'll do a scan.' Nigel puts the scanner on my left side where the pain is and I wait, fully expecting a huge cancerous tumour to come into view. 'No ... it's completely normal. The right side is fine, too. Let's do some blood tests to be sure.'

The blood tests are normal. A repeat scan is normal. But still I feel unwell.

'I've been quite depressed,' I tell Nigel. 'Maybe that's why I'm so worried about cancer. Perhaps I'm just focusing on the bad stuff in my life.'

'Maybe, but let's do a couple more ultrasound scans to be sure.'

The scans are normal and Nigel is so kind about everything. I begin to feel as if I am going crazy. I cannot shake off this constant feeling that everything is under threat. I am so aware of the Limpet lurking in my past, waiting for everything to be okay, lulling me into complacency … and then ambushing my life. I decide to do some research.

In the hospital library I come across some medical literature on the long-term psychological effects of childhood cancer. It is the story of the sword of Damocles. As I read it, I begin to laugh. All these years I have pictured the sword above my head, ready to fall at any moment, and here it is, written in black and white. I picture the vivid scene of Damocles sitting on a cushion at a splendid banquet. Above his head, he knows, there hangs a sword, freshly sharpened and perfectly positioned to split his skull in two. At any moment the hair suspending the sword could snap, just when the best and tastiest dish is about to be served, delivering the fatal, untimely blow. Damocles Syndrome, it says. Living with the constant awareness of death, growing up with it, blaming it for everything. Yes, that is exactly how it is. I take out my pen and start writing. I record the way in which the Limpet has affected me – and afterwards it feels so good. I have acknowledged the shadow cast over my life.

Three months later, in January 1999, I read my article in print in the *British Medical Journal*. 'The sharp edge of Damocles', I called it.

'You know, I can't believe how convinced I was last year that my cancer was back.'

'I know,' says Richard, 'but I guess after Bethany was born you must have been thinking a lot about your future, watching the children grow up and planning for them.'

'Well, I've decided now. I can't waste any more time dwelling on that stupid Limpet. Writing that article helped me put it in perspective. Let's face it – it's more likely that I will be run over by a bus than my cancer returning after sixteen years.'

'Margaret, I'm not going to be able to make it into work – I'm not at all well,' I tell my secretary.

'You sound really rough. What's happened to your voice?'

'Not sure – I can hardly talk. I feel awful, too.'

'You'd better get yourself to the doctor then.'

'I'm going tonight.'

It is 11 February 1999. I think I've picked up a chest infection. My asthma is really going off, despite increasing all my inhalers. It's never been this bad before, I tell my GP.

'And I also coughed up a bit of blood. My asthma has got worse since my little girl was born. I've had a couple of infections. I know it's probably not linked, but I had an osteosarcoma in 1983, so when I saw the blood – well, I panicked a bit. I hope you don't think I'm over-reacting.'

'No, you did the right thing. I'm sure it's just the infection. But I think we had better send you for a chest X-ray to be on the safe side.' He listens to my chest. 'Gosh, you are very wheezy. What are you taking?'

'I've doubled up my inhalers – both the ventolin and the steroid – but it hasn't really made any difference.'

'Okay. Quadruple them, take these antibiotics and attend for your chest X-ray. Come back if there are any more problems.'

I leave the surgery and get into the car. I stuff the X-ray form into the glove compartment. 'Haven't got time for that,' I think to myself. I push away all thoughts of Limpets and swords.

Over the next few days I wait impatiently to get better, but I don't. I get worse, and soon I am back at the surgery.

'I'm still no better. My asthma is just the same.'

The doctor looks at the charts of my peak-flow measurements which I use to monitor my asthma. 'They are right down,' he comments. 'They have never been this low, have they?'

'No, never. Not even when I've had an infection.'

'Right. I'll have to start you on steroid tablets, a new type of inhaler and some different antibiotics … was your X-ray clear?'

'I haven't been …'

The doctor looks at me. 'Why not?'

'Well … I guess I haven't had the time …' Of course I could have made time but, deep down, I don't want to go. I don't want to know, you see. I would rather be in glorious denial. 'I suppose I have been avoiding it …'

'Mary, you can't avoid it. We need to know if there is a problem in your lungs. I'm sure it will be clear, but with your history …'

The unspoken words hang in the air alongside Damocles' sword.

'Okay. I'll go tomorrow.'

Tomorrow arrives and I cannot face it.

'I'll take the steroids for three days and then I know I will be better,' I convince myself. But three days later I am not better. I am even worse. The steroids have made no difference at all, which I know is very much out of the ordinary. I head off to the hospital with a heavy heart.

'It will be something simple,' I tell myself. 'It can't be anything else. Not after all these years.'

I make my way to the X-ray department and a kindly volunteer shows me to the poky changing-room. 'Now, you must strip off to the waist and put on this gown. Take off your cross from around your neck.'

In days gone by I would have interrupted her impatiently and said: 'Yes, I know, I've had hundreds.' But this time I don't. I feel strangely comforted by her helpful advice. I don't want to be a competent doctor. I would rather be a helpless child. I need somebody to take charge and guide me through the horrible journey. But the X-ray will be clear, I know.

'Breathe in!' calls the radiographer from behind the protective screen. I do so, wondering idly how many times my chest has been zapped by radiation. Maybe it's caused some damage. No, I can't think like that. I remember Dr Gupta, who would come into the room full of smiles. 'It's clear, Mary!' he would say cheerfully and then go on to ask me about my medical studies. This time it will be the same.

I sit in the tiny cubicle, awaiting the result. I hear the radiographer moving along the row of cubicles. 'It's clear,' he says to each lady, and then passes to the next.

He misses my door and goes on to the lady on my right. 'It's clear,' he says to her and continues down the line. I sit in the cubicle looking at the door. He's missed me out. Why? Why has he missed me out? Stupid man. There is a picture on the door of a stork carrying a baby. 'Are you pregnant?' it says. 'Tell the radiographer before your X-ray.' It's on all the doors. I've seen the sign every time. Why do they use a stupid picture of a stork? Do they think women are all stupid? Just draw a womb and a baby and tell it how it is – not a stork, for crying out loud. I am just so angry with that man because he has gone down the line and missed me out. He has probably done it on purpose to wind me up. I hate this cubicle. It's so small. How can they expect you to feel calm in here? Maybe I'll just smash the door down and yell at him: look, come back, you stupid moron, tell me it's okay and let me go home. But no he carries on down the line telling everyone else to go home apart from me and it's not fair. I try not to cry. I feel very left out. I have to stay here like some child kept in for detention when I haven't done anything wrong. Why should I be kept in? Why does everybody pick on me? Stupid man and stupid cubicle and stupid stork and stupid bloody stupid evil bastard stupid Limpet. Get lost everybody get lost and leave me alone.

'Dr Self?' enquires the radiographer. I compose myself and open the door.

'Yes? Is there a problem?'

'Dr Self, has anybody ever noted anything on your X-ray before?'

I breathe a sigh of relief – so that's it! They have noticed my first rib is missing. I had it taken out five years ago because it was compressing my blood vessels.

'Yes,' I relax straight away. 'I had surgery. My first left rib is absent.'

'We noticed that … No, what I meant to say – has anybody ever spotted any other abnormality?'

'Abnormality? What kind of abnormality?' I am not prepared for this.

'Well, perhaps if I show you it would be easier.' The radiographer holds the X-ray aloft. 'This is the problem, just here …'

'See here, Little Lady, this is the problem, just here …'

I look this time with my doctor's eye.

And I see it: white, hard and perfectly round, a tumour, a coin lesion, sitting in my lung.

'A penny,' I think to myself. 'It looks just like a penny.' I swallow hard, peer more closely and I know instantly what it is. I recognize this alien. I have seen it before. Without a shadow of a doubt, this is the Limpet's child. An invasion in my lung. I recognize an enemy when I see one and I have been here before. Now I'm battle-trained but I'm still scared to … Death. Oh God. I'm dying. My heart is pounding in my chest and my pulse keeps time – 180 beats per minute down the worst-case scenario. My breath comes in sharp bursts and the voice of the radiographer recedes into the distance. Before I know it, I am planning my funeral, deciding what hymns will be sung, filling the church with yellow tulips and choosing who I should ask to speak about me. I am facing the Limpet again. Oh my God, after all these years. I was right – I knew I was right, I knew there was something wrong with my body. Finally the bloody Limpet evil bastard has won.

'Would you like to speak with one of the doctors?' The radiographer looks at me. I could be wrong. It's a long time since I set eyes on the Limpet and yet it seems it was only yesterday.

'Yes, that would be very helpful, but I would like to get my husband. He works upstairs on the intensive care unit. I'll go and get him, we'll be back in a few minutes.'

158

I try to leave the department with composure. I walk along the corridors as if I am in a dream. My mind searches frantically for alternatives. Nothing recurs after sixteen years. But what else could it be? Richard will know. He will take one look at it and explain.

I walk down the corridor of intensive care. I see my friend Sabine in the distance.

'Hi, Mary. Are you looking for Richard? He's anaesthetizing in theatre.'

'Sabine,' I say, in a complete panic. 'There's a shadow on my chest X-ray.'

She knows the implication. 'Okay. Pauline, take Mary to the coffee room while I track Richard down.'

Pauline, the ward clerk, takes me into the common room and makes me a hot drink. 'So you're Mary,' she says. 'We've heard a lot about you. I've seen pictures of your lovely kids.'

My kids?

Oh no my kids.

Yes, my kids are beautiful and they are so special I waited so long for them and I never thought I would have them. Why, God, why, why are You taking me away from them? After all I went through to get Bethany, I can't believe You want this for me. She won't have a mother, she won't even remember me, You can't do this to her, You can't do this to me.

'Richard will be here soon,' says Pauline. 'Sabine is taking over his case.'

Richard. How will he cope? He will never get over it. I am his life. I am his world. He will never recover from losing me. God, You can't do this to all these people who would be so hurt, so lost, don't let it be cancer please don't let it be cancer.

And then I see Richard strolling down the corridor, looking very much the doctor. I rush up to him and my words tumble out.

'Richard, there is a shadow on my X-ray – it doesn't look like a met but it does look like the Limpet, or at least how I remember it looked. What can it be? It looks just like a cannon ball – maybe it's a secondary from something else, maybe in my kidney or ovary or something but maybe it's nothing, maybe it's benign, do you think it's benign?'

'Hold on, Mary. What does it look like?'

'Come and see it.'

'You say it is heavily calcified?'

'Yes, it's white. And about the size of a penny.'

159

'So it isn't very big?'

'Well, it may not be big but it's still in my bloody lung.'

'And whereabouts is it? Base, apex, middle, hilum?'

'Base. Right base. Out near the edge.'

'Well, that is a very unusual place for a tumour. Maybe it's TB or something like that.'

'Brilliant. Yes, of course. I'm sure that is what it is. But come and look anyway.'

We arrive back in X-ray. Richard waves to a couple of people he knows and meets a fellow doctor. I trudge behind them as they discuss another case. I feel about sixteen again, trailing along behind my dad. It's safer to be small because then you don't have to know the truth.

We see the consultant. 'Hello, I've just been having a look at your wife's X-ray.' He doesn't talk to me and I'm glad because then I can carry on pretending that the Penny does not belong to me. He puts it up on the illuminated box and taps it.

'This is very unusual,' he says in a calm voice. I feel angry again. I don't want to be unusual. He actually sounds pleased it is unusual. Oh, I get it. He wants to show it round his colleagues and they will all have a clever discussion about it and forget this X-ray has an owner. She is thirty-three and has two kids or don't you care about that?

'I think it's benign,' he says, smiling at me in a reassuring manner. I would like to hit him. It's okay for him, sitting there. It's not his chest X-ray. And what if it isn't benign, hey, what if it's malignant? What if it's the Limpet's offspring or another breed of Limpet, then what? I'll tell you what, I get to die, that's what, and you just sit there pontificating on my X-ray. Benign? I want to scream no no no you are wrong you are so wrong this is a nasty evil bastard in my lung, I know, I just know.

'It is so heavily calcified,' the radiologist continues. 'And sixteen years down the line – with an osteosarcoma – it would be unheard of for it to be a secondary.'

'Yes, and it is very peripheral,' adds Richard. 'A secondary would be more central, wouldn't it?'

'Generally, yes. But with Mary's history we need to check it out.'

'What do you think it is?' I ask the radiologist, hesitantly.

'Well, I can't commit myself, and you will need further tests, but I think it is a calcified hamartoma, which is a rare and benign tumour.'

I feel strangely detached from the conversation, as if I am suspended above the room and looking down on this little group of doctors intelligently discussing a chest X-ray. I watch myself nodding and agreeing but my mind is flying up high and saying no no you're wrong. In a flash I recall this happening to me a lot. I would leave my body. My mind would go flying away. I used to think I was going crazy.

'Acute stress reaction. I had an out-of-body experience in there. It was bizarre,' I tell Richard afterwards. 'But he did say it was probably benign, didn't he?'

'Yes, he did. He said it was probably a hamartoma and you need a CT scan. You will most likely end up having a biopsy, too.'

'How will they do that?'

'Not sure. He seemed to think they could stick a needle into it under X-ray control. But let's wait and see what the scan shows.'

The following day is my birthday, 20 February 1999. I am thirty-four years old. Sixteen years ago I celebrated my birthday with the Limpet in my life and now I have the second generation – the Penny in my lung.

Adam comes racing into my room as the day begins: 'Happy birthday to you! Happy birthday to you ...' he enthusiastically sings. 'I've made you a card, Mum!' and he produces a six-year-old's creation of stickers and glitter. 'I've got some flowers for you! Close your eyes ... surprise!' He hands me a bunch of yellow tulips. I smile and kiss him but my eyes fill with tears. He is so blissfully unaware of the troubling news and I wish I could be, too. 'Daddy says we are going to the beach today.' It is a very sunny day but freezing cold. 'It's your birthday surprise – and I have bought you a cake,' he whispers, 'but don't tell Dad I told you!'

I wrap my arms around him. 'Give me a cuddle then!' I say. 'A special one for my birthday.' I hold him close and smell the sweetness of his skin. 'You're the best mummy in the world!' says Adam and I put my face in his soft hair and ask myself why? How can my life be threatened by such darkness now? Adam is only six and Bethany only one. I bargain with God. 'I'll do anything – anything! Just don't take me away from them. They need me. It's not fair on them – don't You see, God? I'm sure You must. Just give me until they are a little older and can do without me. Please. Let the Penny be benign.'

And so we head to the beach on the brightest February day I can remember. We go to Weston-super-Mare because there are donkeys. Bethany has never seen a donkey. She has never seen sand. When we arrive, Adam jumps out of the car and runs down to the beach.

161

Bethany toddles along after him. Her feet reach the soft sand and she looks down, so puzzled. She stoops to touch and it sticks to her fingers. She wipes her hands clean on Adam's coat. I laugh to see my daughter discovering sand. It is such a simple pleasure. I feel ecstatic and I hoard the joy.

We all laugh as Bethany spots the donkeys and squeals in amazement. Richard lifts her up to stroke an ear. Adam is set to go on his first donkey ride. He waves as they trot up the beach. I lift my head and breathe the salty air in deeply. The cold wind catches my eyes and they water. It is as if the whole scene is in slow motion. I need to experience every sensation more deeply. 'Treasure these moments,' I tell myself. 'Squeeze every drop of joy from them, every last drop. Live, love, laugh and drink it all in – just in case they do not come again.'

For I know this is a moment in harbour. This is the calm before the storm. This day with my children is a memory to sustain me through the dark days I know are ahead.

I remember how I used to store up my good times like a squirrel gathering for winter. I was seventeen then. I was naïve and raw, untutored in life. But how I wanted to live that life. 'I want to make the most of what little time I may have,' I remember telling my parents. What pain they must have felt, I now understand, as I watch my own children playing happily. Back then I was a girl on the threshold of becoming a woman. I was a girl with ambitions and hopes and dreams. So many things, it seemed, were about to be taken from me. I shudder as I remember the moment I contemplated life without my left leg. Not just my form but my function destroyed. I thought I would be denied life itself. And if I were to escape the shadow of death I never imagined that I would be loved, that I would learn to laugh again. Yet there were moments of happiness even within that terror. Every experience was hoarded carefully, like pretty shells to be gathered and put on display. Things I could say I had done, achieved. There were moments of intense and exquisite beauty, magnified a hundredfold, a thousandfold, because they were lived against the blackest of backgrounds. I smile as I recall tasting my first garlic bread – truly delicious! I remember the daffodils in the little park at the end of the road, their yellow cheerfulness defying the bitter cold. For my collection, I gathered a glass of red wine sparkling in a crystal glass and a rainbow shimmering over a waterfall, the soft swish of cream taffeta against my skin and the warmth of my sisters' bodies holding me close. And then I collected my

A levels – the centrepiece of my display! Now I understand how I could know happiness amid despair. I once said the dark days contained some of the happiest moments of my life and now I understand why. The brightness of pure gold shining against black velvet. My senses sharpened keenly against a cruel stone of pain.

Before there is an opportunity to have my CT scan, I get sick again. Even though I am on maximum doses of my inhalers, high doses of steroids and double doses of antibiotics, my asthma gets worse. One morning I am resting in bed and I get even wheezier. I take all my inhalers and they don't work. I take them again and they still don't work. 'Try not to worry,' I tell myself, 'asthma gets worse with anxiety.' But I keep thinking about the Penny in my lung and know it is responsible. Only an evil and malicious Penny would produce such severe symptoms. 'Asthma can be fatal,' I remember. I measure my peak flow. It is only 200. It is normally 500. Less than half – I know I need help. I call the surgery and try to explain. I'm on my own – I can't breathe – I'm on maximum treatment. Asthma can kill you.

I am admitted to the University Hospital of Wales as an emergency: acute severe asthma. I am a seasoned patient. I have spent years of my life perfecting the art. For the first few hours I adjust to the sick role. I tell the nurse my story, let her measure my blood pressure and my peak flows, hold out my wrist obediently for my identity bracelet. She shows me how to administer my nebulized medication and then she stops suddenly.

'What am I doing? You're a doctor, I don't need to tell you!'

'Oh no!' I reply. 'Don't tell them that – I won't get any peace.'

But it isn't just that. I don't want to be a doctor now. I reject the professional-mother-of-two image and opt for regression – temporarily. I want to curl up and feel sorry for myself. I cuddle my little boy's teddy and I am soothed by the voices of the older ladies on the ward. I am quietened by their hushed whispers. They discuss my condition, my doctors and the manner of my arrival. Their concern and clichés comfort me, for we are all in this together, our control removed and our dignity dented. We are all in a state of helpless dependency. The curtains are drawn around me and I spend a therapeutic ten minutes analysing them. Hospital curtains are always the same – colours that clash and lots of holes. There are big gaps at the top where the curtain hooks are missing and I feel annoyed that the symmetry is spoiled. They look lopsided. Lopsided …

I see the feet I dread beneath the hem of the curtain. I often draw the curtains around me. They are a barrier between them and me. The other patients are old and dying. I am young and alive – just about. When I am behind the curtains nothing can hurt me. Except the feet I see beneath the hem and the world I see when they are pulled back. I always know who the feet belong to. Dr Tan-Shoes wears horrible shoes. They are the colour of my bedpan contents on a Methotrexate day. He always wears trousers that are too short and don't match. And I'm scared of him and his dish with the needles in, although they look so pretty. I'm scared of the yellow poison in the drip. I'm scared of my hair falling out and my ovaries shrivelling … but most of all I'm scared of dying. I do not know how to die. Dr Tan-Shoes holds power over my life in his kidney-shaped dish. So I smile at him, even though I hate him. I keep still while he sticks the fiery sharp needles into my arms and I hold back my tears. I hold back so much of myself. When I draw back the curtains I have to be meek and gentle and mild, like Jesus, and then the priests will be very pleased with me. I will help to convert maybe hundreds of people. And then there will be a reason – because I do need a reason. It cannot be for nothing, this pain, this mutilation. And if I convert loads of people then maybe God will be very pleased with me because of doing lots of good things. And then I will get better and I won't have to think about cancer and dying any more …

My best friend, Eleanor, draws back the curtains. She works as a nurse manager in the University Hospital of Wales, where I have been admitted. We first met when Richard and I moved to Cardiff in 1995 but I have only got to know her well over the last year. We love singing together in the worship group at church. Ellie is a few years older than me and a lot wiser. She is always very calm and constant – a great person to have around in a crisis. I think we get on because she has known life be pretty tough, too. She fought her way through troubled times as a single mum, bringing up two young children, before she married Ian eight years ago. She shares my stubborn determination to overcome. And she has that same desire to have a faith that demon-strates itself in real and practical ways. Ellie would help anybody who was in trouble. She seems to have this huge capacity to love – but it is a tough and sensible love. Sometimes Ellie despairs of my intensely passionate emotions. I think I make her laugh a lot. Recently, I have made her cry a lot, too.

'Hello,' she says. 'I told you I would visit.'

'Ellie – I was so scared. I thought I was back there. You know, back being seventeen again. I thought I was wearing the mask again – pretending I feel okay when all I feel is scared.'

'Hey, it's okay to feel scared. God knows how you feel. But you also know He is never going to leave you on your own. You don't have to be scared because He has you safe in the palm of His hand.'

'I'm so scared the cancer is back again. My mind keeps running away from me, running away to the past when I was so very frightened. Then it runs forward to the future and that terrifies me, too.'

'Okay, I know. But you need to stay in the present. We need to get you through today. Tomorrow can worry about itself.'

'Tell me I'm not there any more – seventeen, dying and facing the unknown.'

'You know you're not. You are Mary: thirty-four years old, doctor, wife, mother and a strong and mature Christian. Whatever you face, you are not alone. You will get through it with God on your side and your family and friends who love you.'

A week later I have been discharged and am waiting with Richard in Llandough Hospital to see Dr Smith, who specializes in lung tumours. Now at last I will know the truth. The clinic is a depressing place. I am surrounded by other patients, all of whom appear to be very ill. Most of them are wearing oxygen masks and several are painfully thin. The man opposite me is panting and puffing. His lips are a deep shade of blue and every breath seems to be an effort. I can see the outline of his bones, the skin stretched tautly over them like a wigwam. Many of the patients peer curiously at me. The notice board is covered with leaflets announcing various cancer helplines and I feel an overwhelming urge to run away and never return.

'Dr Self … Come in. I'm Dr Smith.' He gestures towards a large group of medical students. 'Do you mind if they remain in the room? Your case is most unusual.'

'No, not at all.'

Dr Smith reads the referral letter and then asks me more questions about the bone tumour and my recent asthma problems. I tell my story and hand him the X-rays. He pins them up on the light box and we all peer at the Penny.

'Mr Griffiths,' he says, addressing one of the students, 'kindly tell us what you see. And meantime, Louise, take Dr Self to the examination room and settle her on the couch.' I guess Louise must be a third-year. Despite my ten years' medical experience, I feel strangely unsure of myself and shy. I get flustered as she hands me a gown. In the background I can hear Mr Griffiths stumbling with the X-ray.

'A coin lesion ... right lung ... past history of osteosarcoma.'

'And the likely sites of spread for an osteosarcoma? Anybody?'

'Lung, brain, liver,' answers a female voice.

'Correct.'

I feel terrified as I contemplate the awful prospect of other Pennies. I am so distracted that I have trouble getting my gown on.

'Here, let me help you. I'll tie the back for you,' says Louise. I lean forward and let her take over. I am a patient now, another case and an interesting one at that. This doctor is a specialist on Pennies and I know he thinks it is a secondary.

Louise hands me a glass of water. I take it and see my hand is trembling. My mouth is so dry. I look around, not seeing anything except the image in my mind of the Penny on my X-ray.

Dr Smith examines me, then sends the students away for a coffee break and looks at me seriously.

'Well, Dr Self, we obviously need to biopsy this tumour.'

'I'm so worried – what do you think it is? I mean, it's seventeen years since my bone tumour ... surely it couldn't spread so late on?'

'Yes, it would be most unusual. However, with your history I think we must assume this is malignant until proved otherwise.'

There is a long and heavy silence while Richard and I take in these words.

'So what type of biopsy are you thinking of?'

'The tumour is calcified – it would be like stone. I just don't think it would be possible to obtain a sample with a needle. It has to be an open biopsy.'

'So that would mean an operation?'

Richard looks at me warily. 'Mary, Dr Smith means you need a thoracotomy.'

'A thoracotomy ...'

I have seen thoracotomies in my time as an anaesthetist. There is nothing more fearsome. The rib cage is opened through the back, the lung collapsed and the tumour removed. The operation is long and very painful.

'I am going to refer you to a cardio-thoracic surgeon. Your asthma is still very severe, so I'm not sure if he will be happy to operate with your lungs as they are. That is up to the anaesthetist. Your breathing is terrible but I'm sure the tumour is making things worse.'

I look at the X-ray. The Penny looks so small, so innocent. It even looks quite pretty, all perfectly round. I cannot believe my chest is going to be cut in half and prised apart because of it. I feel the sting of tears as I contemplate what lies ahead. Oh God, it is too much. And yet there is still more.

'Dr Self,' adds Dr Smith gently. 'I think we should check out the other likely sites of spread before we do a thoracotomy under such circumstances.'

'What do you mean? I'm fine – I know I'm fine.'

'We really need to scan your brain as a priority.'

'Why?' I almost yell at him, feeling angry at him for bringing up a topic more horrible than I can imagine.

'Well, if there is anything in your brain …'

'You mean, basically there would be no point operating.'

'Your prognosis would then be so poor …'

My brain, please not in my brain. Fainting and fits and half-heard whispers. Dr Jimmy outside my room and somebody shaking me and my muscles hurting all over. And fear and madness so great that all I want to do is to slice into my body with sharp, sharp glass and rid myself of all the evil the Limpet brings. A Limpet in my brain – that would be worse than death. I would turn into some drooling, incontinent skeleton slumped in a wheelchair. A living death. So please, God, please – not my brain.

The following day I attend for my brain scan. I am shown into the room. The radiologist chats to me about my children and my job as she helps me onto the couch. She lifts my head and positions it in the little rubber cushion. 'I used to call this machine the magic Polo mint,' I tell her.

'We still call it that for the children,' she replies and then with a friendly wave leaves the room. I am terrified – but not of the scan. I have lain here maybe half a dozen times over the years. I no longer need to call the scanner by a pet name. Hospitals, scanners, needles and tests are as familiar as the air that I breathe. No, I am terrified of what might be in my brain. I am terrified that another Limpet or another Penny will be discovered there. For then I know there will be no hope.

'Be not afraid!' I whisper to myself. I remember whispering it so many years ago. God will heal me. He has healed me before. I know I can face the surgery but God I don't know if I can face a met in my brain. Oh God I am asking You to spare me this. I need to know peace in this. I place it in Your hands, Lord. I need to feel Your presence with me now, here. Strengthen me for whatever lies ahead.

The scan is clear. My brain has no secondaries – no Limpet and no Penny. The surgery can go ahead.

Several days later I arrive in the cardio-thoracic unit. I introduce myself to the ward clerk and see my name written in her book. 'Removal of pulmonary metastasis – thoracotomy.' I have already been stereotyped. I am dying until proved otherwise.

Richard arrives on the ward a few minutes after I do. A doctor looks up from the desk. 'Hi, Richard!' he says. 'Which patient have you come to see?'

'Actually, this is my wife.'

'Oh, yes. I've seen the X-rays. Fascinating. Most unusual.'

I want to scream: 'Yes, I know I'm interesting, fascinating and unusual – but I have a life, I have two children and I just want to be plain boring. I want to be the common-or-garden variety of case. I don't want to be rare.'

I am shown to the high-dependency section. Of the four beds, one is occupied by a lady who has just come back from theatre, presumably having had a thoracotomy. She is sitting upright and the nurses are fixing her oxygen mask. She has two big chest drains inserted in her wounds and they are already half full of blood. She is moaning in pain. Two nurses attend to her and I see the scale of the surgery I am to undergo. I unpack my bag and arrange the photographs of my children so I can see them easily. I stick my little scripture cards to my locker and put on my nightdress. Now I am a patient. I lie on my bed and try to blot out the noise of the lady moaning and the constant hiss of the mask helping her breathe.

Dr Vaughan, the anaesthetist, comes to assess my breathing. I know Dr Vaughan – in fact, he has taught me. He sits on the edge of the bed and greets me. 'Mary,' he says, and his tone of voice says it all. 'Tell me what has been happening.' So I tell Dr Vaughan about the asthma and the tumour and how frightened I feel.

'You're the same as everybody else then, Mary. Every patient is scared of this operation. You are not immune because you are a doctor. Be brave! You are in good hands.'

I wait while he reads the letter in my notes from Dr Smith. I know what it says – I sneaked a look at my notes while I was undressing.

Dr Vaughan sighs. I know he is upset; I can see his eyes are too bright. I know Dr Smith is pretty certain this tumour is a lung secondary. I suppose I will know soon enough but first I have to survive the surgery. Dr Vaughan has to get me through it.

'Well, Mary,' Dr Vaughan says. 'Your asthma is very bad at the moment but I don't think we can improve it so we will go ahead. There is a risk to the surgery but we have to get this tumour out of your lung. Do you have any questions?'

'What about the pain. I know it can be awful after this operation.'

'I would like to suggest an epidural. It will help your pain and enable you to cough and that is vital after this type of surgery.' As he leaves, he gives me a hug.

Early next morning I am woken to shower and prepare for surgery. As I put on the white gown and paper pants I feel tearful. Half my life ago I joined battle as the Limpet waged war on my body …

'Mary Clewlow!' A loud voice shouts down the corridor. I spin round. I am not used to Mr Peach being cross. 'What are you doing, walking down the corridor in bare feet? You have just showered for your operation. Think of all those germs on the floor!' He wags his finger at me in mock anger. 'Go on … back you go, Little Lady, and put those feet under the shower again!'

'You're joking?'

'I am not! I don't want any horrid germs in my operating theatre. Back you go!' So I trudge down the corridor. The floor is cold and slippery beneath my toes. I stand and stick my feet under the shower and scrub them with pink, smelly antiseptic. The nurse brings me some sterile paper overshoes. I walk back up the corridor and climb onto the bed. It was the last time I washed my left foot, the last time I walked on my own two legs …

I am sleepy as I am wheeled down another long and draughty corridor. Richard walks at my side. I recall my dad's long stride and how small and helpless I felt. Richard bends to kiss me as we arrive at the theatre. 'See you when you wake up. I love you.' He slips my favourite scripture card under my pillow – Psalm 23.

'I love you, too.'

Dr Vaughan is in the anaesthetic room with my friend Sabine. I am to have my epidural put in while I am awake, to ensure it is working

169

before I go off to sleep. I have a first drip inserted and then sit up on the trolley while Sabine holds my hand.

'The Lord is my Shepherd, there is nothing I shall want ...'

'Okay, Mary, keep nice and still – this is the epidural needle.'

'He makes me lie down in green pastures. He leads me beside still waters. He restores my soul ...'

'It's in. I'm going to give you a test dose. Let's lie you down.'

'I feel numb – my legs are all heavy.'

'Breathe through the mask. Slowly – that's it. It's just oxygen.'

'It's okay, Mary, squeeze my hand. Dr Vaughan is putting the drip in now.'

'He guides me in paths of righteousness – for His name's sake.'

'Mary, this is a big dose of Fentanyl coming now. It will make you feel drowsy.'

'Even though I walk through the valley of the shadow of death ... Whoah, that's nice!'

'Okay, Mary?'

'Oh yes! I'm terrific! Sabine! What are you doing here? The lights are moving around.'

'It's just the Fentanyl working.'

'I will fear no evil.'

'Mary, you're going to drift off in a few seconds.'

'For You are with me.'

'Are you with me? Mary? Mary?'

'With me. You are with me ...'

A face. Go way face.

'Hello, Mary. You've had your operation.'

A soft female voice breaks into my sleep. I hear the high beep beep of a hundred machines. Where are the noises coming from? I try to speak and look around. I can't move, I am so weak, I am made out of jelly. I am in a strange place. A big white empty room. I hurt. I hurt so much and I am so tired and there is stuff in my mouth. Blood. Something sticks in my mouth. A sucker. The woman holds an ice cube on my tongue and I let the drops go in my mouth. It is lovely. There are tubes everywhere, coming out of my body in all directions. Another awakening. I remember other awakenings. The splint. The first time there was a splint. The second time there was no leg. But there are always tubes and there is always fear and always pain.

'Mary, you're in intensive care. It's Thursday morning. You had your operation yesterday.'

A black hole. I've been in a black hole.

'Richard?'

'Is on his way in.'

Sleep, I sleep. It feels like hours and then Richard is whispering in my ear. 'It's okay. It's benign. I just spoke to the surgeon.'

'I can't believe it …' Sleep again. Sleep for ever now that it's okay …

Another place. It's different. Dark and shadowy. Nobody here apart from me. Curtains. Flowers big flowers. Enormous like tangerine trees and yes they are orange and green. The curtains are drawn. He can't get me. Nobody can get me. The curtains are drawn and the cancer is gone. Then I see a giant peeping over the top of the curtain. I laugh. What are you doing there? He is walking round the curtains trying to find a way in. Why? He looks quite friendly. Tall and thin. I can't see his face. Then his friend arrives and they stand and talk about me. Not yet they say. Not yet and I begin to feel scared so I look at the dancing flowers instead and they are so bright, so orange …

'Mary, it's Cheryl.' I open my eyes to see a friend from church. She is a nurse on the ward. 'Here, I've brought you a drink. Sip through the straw. I hear you had a rough night.'

'I had these terrible dreams. And weird hallucinations.'

'It's the side-effects of the Fentanyl in your epidural. And also because of the steroids and the inhalers we are giving you. It often happens after a thoracotomy. How is your pain?'

'Not too bad. The epidural is working well.'

'Well, you have two chest drains in and your drip. The central line into your neck is coming out today, and you have your bladder catheter until your epidural comes out. And you must keep your oxygen mask on. The chest physio will be along to help you with your coughing and breathing exercises.'

She helps me wash and I feel a little more in reality. She explains that for several weeks I will have to sit up most of the time to help my lungs function. As the day passes, the weakness and tiredness wear off and I am able to move around the bed a little more freely. By evening I am drinking cups of tea and managing to eat a little. The physiotherapist visits and teaches me how to breathe deeply and helps me with my coughing. This will help my lung expand back to normal. I tell the physiotherapist I will cough as much as she wants! All that matters is that I get out of here and go home. My tumour is benign and I can carry on with my life. I can see my precious children grow up! I will see the millennium after all!

Later a middle-aged man is pushed into the room on a trolley. He has just returned from theatre. The nurses draw the curtains round him and I hear the news from the operating theatre.

'He has had his whole lung taken out – pneumonectomy. Frozen section shows a large squamous cell carcinoma, I'm afraid. All the lymph nodes were involved. The surgeons are talking to the family now.'

I feel guilty – guilty that my tumour is benign and his is cancer. I am going to survive but he is going to die from his Limpet. A few hours later his family visit. I guess the two ladies are his wife and daughter. They sit there holding his hands. I pretend not to notice them crying. Inside now the guilt has passed and I just feel overwhelming relief that it is not me this time. With a sickening lurch I realize I am glad because the cancer belongs to somebody else.

But it belonged to me half my life ago. It was bad news then. News doesn't come much worse. I remember the guilt I felt then. I remember thinking the cancer was my fault. I thought God was punishing me for all the bad things I had done. I felt guilty to be causing everybody so much unhappiness and I remember trying to hide my fear and pain. When the first and second miracles failed I blamed myself. Guilt, there was so much guilt.

I talk it over with Ellie when she visits later.

'I used to think it was God punishing me,' I tell her. 'You know – I wasn't trying hard enough or had done bad things.'

'But now you know God loves you. He has given you a new life and you can bin the guilt. The God who gave us Jesus isn't going to punish you.'

'I used to think being healed was a reward for the amount of good things I did. Now I see it is free. If God wants to heal me, then He will. He will just do it. I don't have to earn it. And if He doesn't …'

'Yes? What if He doesn't?'

'Well, that would be awful – but I know He would have something better for me. So if He doesn't heal me, then I can accept that, too. But the tumour is benign so I'm going to be okay now!'

As night falls, the dreams and terror return. I am back to strange sounds and sights. I awake in the night gasping and panicking. I have slipped down the pillows and it is very difficult to breathe. I turn my head to the window. A nurse is sitting quietly, filling in some charts. I feel safe. The phone rings and she leaves the room. As soon as she does, I hear whispering. It is the two giants again. I cannot see them but I can hear them. There she is they say. We can get her soon. What shall we do this time though? They whisper together and I cannot quite hear what they are saying but I know it is fearful whatever they are plotting. My heart beats loudly and I turn over. She is trying to ignore us says one of them. He has a Scouse accent. She thinks we won't notice her if she doesn't look at us. Suddenly they are blowing on my back over my wound. Then I feel their hands pulling at my dressing. Shall we get her? Shall we get her? They are giggling and laughing. Shall we put them in? I hear a clink of metal. Coins it's coins they are putting pennies inside my wound into my lung. Quickly I turn over and the giants retreat to the corner. Let's just watch they say until she falls asleep and then we can put them in. We can get her when she is asleep. So I don't sleep. I stay awake just in case they get me and their incessant whispering drives me crazy but it is better than falling asleep. There is music playing. It's coming out of the smoke alarm. The music is funny and it is laughing. It's the laughing policeman. The giants begin to dance and then I can see they have a seagull chained to the window and the seagull is dancing too. The world, I think, is going crazy. But still I won't fall asleep. I don't want any more bad pennies. If one of the giants has pennies then maybe he is Judas. I try to see his neck but cannot for he is too tall. The one with the Scouse accent, though, I don't know who he is. Maybe Jesus, but why would Jesus want to hurt me? It's all very confusing. The nurse comes back in and sits down again and I feel safe and drift back to sleep.

I am now four days post-op. My lung is back to normal size and I am coughing and breathing well. The doctors are pleased with my progress. They explain what will happen over the next few days.

'We will take one of your chest drains out today and see whether your lung remains stable. If it does we will take the other drain out tomorrow.'

'What about the epidural? When does that come out?'

'Tomorrow. You will have a fair bit of pain once it does.'

'Well, I can cope with that now I know that the tumour is benign.'

'Yes, we just need to get the histology to confirm.'

'Oh – I don't understand. I thought the histology had been done in theatre. I thought they looked at a specimen during the operation.'

'No. The tumour was too hard to cut up. It's being softened now so we can look at it under the microscope. We will have the results in a few days' time.'

'But I thought it was benign?'

'We're ninety-nine per cent sure it's benign.'

'But not a hundred per cent?'

'Well, as I said. We are ninety-nine per cent sure that this is a hamartoma – a benign tumour. But we have been known to be wrong.'

'What if I am the one per cent?'

'Well, it's not very likely. But, like I said, we could be wrong. If we are then we will refer you to Velindre, the oncology hospital. See you tomorrow.'

They leave and I sit numb with shock. I thought there was no doubt about the nature of the tumour. I thought the pathology was definite. I hadn't realized it was only a ninety-nine per cent chance.

I try to be rational. 'A ninety-nine per cent chance is great, fantastic,' I think.

'But it's not one hundred per cent, is it?'

A chink of fear opens in my mind. I push it away. I look at the photograph of my children on the bedside locker. No, surely, this is the end of the time of testing. I cannot possibly be expected to face more.

The drain is taken out of my wound and the dressing removed. Because it is on my back I am unable to see it, and I am curious. I know the scar will be large. My body has become different again and I would like to see my new form. Although the surgery is not mutilating in the same way as my amputation, I feel self-conscious and changed. Later my friend Ruth visits. As she has been a nurse, I feel she is the right person to help me look at my scar.

'Ruth, I need to see this scar. Will you help me stand in front of the mirror?'

'Yes, of course. Let me move all your tubes so you can get closer.' She sorts out the paraphernalia and helps me manoeuvre closer to the mirror on the wall. 'If you stand and hold on to my shoulders, I'll lift your nightdress for you and also help you balance.'

'Okay, I'm ready.'

She lifts my nightie and I look.

Do you want to see your Little Leg now?

I gasp as I look at the clean but huge wound that splits my ribcage in half.

I had pictured it as bloody and bruised but it is pink and soft and healed. Quite cute, really.

'I can't believe it – it looks like a shark attack. It's so ... so radical. So – well, it looks so macho. It's kind of brutally impressive.'

My new body is not ugly, just different.

'Do you think it looks ugly?'
  'No, truly I don't. It's certainly an eye-catcher. When it's healed you could almost make something daring out of it. Wear high necks and low backs. It's so neat and clean-cut that it is almost ... perfect.'
  I smile and admire my scar again. I quite like the idea of the low-backed dress.

Night-time again. Darkness falls. Terror breaks in quickly. The doctor – I have worked out he is an impostor. He is collaborating with the giants and soon they will succeed with their plan. They have persuaded the doctor to give me something to make me sleep and then they will come and get me. I can hear them. I know they are here. They are whispering again. They are all in it together. Out of the corner of my eye I see them walk past the door. I am so tired – exhausted – but if I sleep they will do terrible things to my body. I'm going to escape. Then I hear a sound. It is coming from behind the wall. It is a growling noise. It's a dog, the giants' dog. It must be hungry by now. Then I am laughing and running, running through fields of orange flowers whose scent is over-powering. They smell of incense and vanilla. I stumble and fall and the dog is upon me and the laughter becomes a high-pitched scream. The flowers are turning red and dying. They are dying and so am I and then I see the dog is gnawing my leg only I can't feel it because I am numb all over. The smell is changing and it is sickly and cloying. I know the smell. It is the smell of blood in the sunshine.

On the doctor's round the following day I mention the strange sights and scenes I am experiencing.

'Yes, it happens after this operation – a mixture of the low oxygen levels and the drugs.'

'It's very frightening. It's so real.'

'Mmm. Today we need to take out your chest drain and your epidural and we need to get you up and about.'

'And the hallucinations?'

'They will pass. Your histology is still not back yet. See you tomorrow.'

One by one the tubes are removed and I am free to move around again. I spend the day going for short walks and practising my breathing exercises. I am determined to recover quickly from the surgery and return home soon to the children. I have missed them so much.

The pain is terrible once the epidural is removed. It feels as if there is a tight hot band around my ribcage. The nurses give me strong painkilling tablets to help lessen it, but the pain is always there, gnawing away in the background. By the end of the day I am very tired.

If he is not a doctor, then who is he? He is here to kill me. Kill me horrifically. He will set the hungry dog on me and it will tear me to pieces. It will rip out my brain and my liver and my soul. It already has my leg and my lung and part of my heart. I will escape. I am leaving this place. It is too scary, too frightening. I think somebody put something in the drugs. They are contaminating my body with miniscule mutant cells. So I put on my leg and out I go. Bye bye, I say to the nurse who is not really a nurse but an experimenter. Get away from me I say to the doctor who is an evil man who infects the world with cancer. Say goodbye to the giants for me. I walk out of the ward to the stairs. Then I hear the dog. They will send it after me. I look around and see the stairwell. This is the fifth floor. Ward Eight is on the second floor. If I threw myself out. If I threw myself down. Hi, Steve! Where's Nigel? We all admire you. He saved my baby. You make us think. He is a proper doctor. You'll get through – we're behind you. Tough baby. Jack, Debbie, Lydia … Mary Mary quite contrary, who's next? It's noisy so noisy get out of my head and I'm running running away from the voices the noise in my head, running away from my mind escaping and my soul flying. I'm in a bathroom. There is a rail. I'm scared so scared of the Limpet. I can't escape and I look at the rail. I look at my dressing gown and take out the cord. I see a chair. My breath is too quick and

176

my heart is exploding with fear and terror. I can hear the giants throwing pennies at the door. I drag the chair over, for they will break down the door and that will be it like Jack's wife. Escape them escape them climb up the beanstalk. Climb on the chair. Put the cord around your neck like a collar. They are knocking on the door. Somebody is knocking on the door. Come out, Mary. Come out. I cannot reach the rail. You're safe. You're safe. I come out – no giants. Judas hasn't won. Sit in this room. Sit for a while. Pretty fish in a tank. Watch them swim. Round and round. The fish is laughing at me. 'Whore,' it says in a bubbly, watery voice, it's talking to me, accusing me, 'whore'. It's my fault, it's all because of me. Kill the fish kill it now. I pick up a cup and throw it at the fish. The cup breaks and I am crying just get rid of this in my head get rid of it. I want it to be quiet. It's okay, Mary, it's okay. I'm going mad. It is Vera, my friend. Take this – it will make you better. The drugs have done this. Come on, this is a lovely drink of tea, raspberry tea. Let me soothe you. Come on, get back on the bed – you're okay. I broke the glass. Don't worry, drink this. Yes, I will, I want to be quiet. Sleepy? Yes sleepy. Sleepy and quiet. At last.

'Ellie. What happened? I feel so weird.'

'You developed a psychosis. Apparently it does happen after major operations. The drugs could also have contributed to it.'

'Oh no,' I groan, 'tell me what I did.'

'You really want to know? You absconded from the ward, claiming all the doctors were impostors, and locked yourself in the bathroom. Then you threw a cup at the fish tank in the dayroom!'

'Is everybody cross at me?'

'Nobody is cross, just concerned. You can't help the fact that you went psychotic. It happens.'

'But why me?'

'Mary, you are on a stack of medication, you have had a horrible operation and you're worrying about the diagnosis. Now, as a psychiatrist, would you say you were a likely candidate?'

'I suppose so, but it's just so embarrassing. I'm not sure I want to relate quite so closely to my patients' illnesses! What happened next?'

'One of the psychiatric nurses managed to get some Haloperidol down you and that knocked you out. Talking of which, you need to take this second dose now. Come on – before you cause any more trouble.'

Soon the doctor arrives. I smile meekly and apologetically at him.

'Hospital seems to be driving you mad, quite literally,' he says. 'I spoke to Richard just now and he can take some time off. So I think we should get you home on Saturday – the day after tomorrow.'

'What did the fish say to you?' laughs Ellie.

'I can't repeat it, but I'll tell you one thing: hallucinations are very frightening. I never want to go through that again. Give me pain any day. At least that is understandable.'

Two days later I am packing my bags and saying goodbye to the nurses.

'I can't believe I'm through it!' I say to Richard. 'And the news is looking good. I know that it is still a one per cent chance, but I'll bet on that.'

'Yes,' agrees Richard. 'Everybody is so positive. If there was any real possibility of this being a secondary, we would know by now.'

Adam has decorated the front door with pictures. A colourful creation of hearts and flowers adorns it.

'Welcome home Mummy!' he has written. It is over a week since I have seen my children and I have missed them so much. As soon as the car pulls up outside the door Adam runs out to greet me.

'I missed you, Mummy! You are the best mummy in the world!' He flings his arms around me and hugs me tightly. Little Bethany toddles after him and we all go inside. I sit down and Bethany tries to climb on my knee. I reach forward and an agonizing pain shoots through my shoulder.

'I'll help you, Mummy!' says Adam and he hauls Bethany onto my knee, smiling broadly at being so grown-up.

'I know,' I reply, burying my head in Bethany's soft, messy curls. And nothing really matters except being here as a family and knowing we are going to be together. I have been looking death in the face for the last two months. I thought the Limpet had won. I cannot believe that, after all the worry, everything has worked out. I am going to see my kids grow up. I am going to make it into the next millennium. I have a future. I'm going to live!

I look at my two precious children – miracles, both of them. 'It's strange really, isn't it?' I say to myself. 'I thought it was a bad penny. I thought my life was over just as theirs had begun. Bad pennies have this habit of turning up at the wrong time, don't they?'

The Penny remains calmly and complacently silent.

God doesn't say much, either.

11

'I don't know what to say, Dr Smith ... I guess, when I didn't hear, I assumed everything was looking good. It's just such a huge shock. To be honest, I had stopped worrying about the results.'

I am still shaking my head in disbelief. I received the phone call yesterday, asking me to attend clinic today. It is now four weeks since my thoracotomy. I have made an excellent recovery from the surgery. My wound has healed nicely, my pain is settling and my asthma completely better. It is May 1999, and I thought I had come to the end of this traumatic episode. Now I see it has only just begun ...

'Well, Little Lady, you must be brave. That old lump – well, it was a nasty old thing.'

'Dr Self, I'm afraid it's not good news.'

'I'm afraid the lump was cancer.'

'I'm afraid the tests showed it is malignant.'

It is an osteosarcoma.

It is a secondary from the original osteosarcoma.

I have bone cancer. I am only seventeen.

I have a secondary in my lung. I am only thirty-four.

I am scared.

I am very scared.

'I am so sorry, Mary. I cannot really give you any more information. As you know, this is out of my area of expertise now.'

'So what happens?'

'I will refer you to one of the oncologists at Velindre. I'm sure they will see you very soon. I do hope things work out for you.'

He shakes my hand and I walk out of his room. Somehow I manage to walk down the corridor and find my way back to Richard, waiting outside. He looks at me and knows straight away. He takes me by the arm and leads me to a bench outside in a small garden area. I sit very still, like a statue. There are some late blossom trees and I stare at them, noticing the perfection of the delicate petals. Two blackbirds are fighting over a worm. One wins and flies off to the branches of a tree. I catch the scent of blossom on the breeze as I turn to look at Richard. Spring is turning into summer. The summer has suddenly become shorter.

'Richard – what are we going to do? It's malignant.'

Richard looks back at me and I see in his eyes the realization that nothing is certain any longer. He puts his arms around me and we hold each other.

'Why? Why now? I don't even know what the prognosis is. Dr Smith didn't know. I have to go to Velindre.'

The blackbird returns, looking for more worms. I think it must have a nest in the tree with two or three fledglings in it.

'What about the children? I can't bear to think of it. They won't even remember me properly. They are so very young.'

'Shh, Mary. We don't know yet what the outlook is, whether there is any treatment …' His voice tails off, for we both know the reality.

'Richard, it's a death sentence. Metastases from a sarcoma – we both know the score.'

'Seventeen years … I can't believe it has happened after so many years. We thought you were cured.'

'Okay – we need to stay calm. We must not panic.'

'Absolutely. We need to keep our heads in all this. We don't know for certain.'

'Maybe it's a mistake? Maybe we should get a second opinion?'

'Yes, we could do that. We need to be strong.'

We sit in silence for a few more minutes. I remember all the anniversaries we have shared, right back to the very first on the Mersey ferry.

180

And all the time the Limpet was just waiting for the most painful moment to attack.

'Richard, I'm sorry,' I say. 'I'm sorry I have brought you all this pain. I'm so sorry,' and then, as I look at him and he shakes his head, I begin to feel the release of tears and cry softly.

'Mary, it's for better, for worse, remember? In sickness and in health.'

'Yes I know,' I sob. 'Till death us do part as well and I don't want to part. I don't want to leave you.'

'I don't want to lose you,' and now Richard is crying too. Everybody stares as they walk past us but I don't care. It is my grief. Our grief is too heavy and one we should not know at thirty-four. We are too young.

'Do you regret marrying me? Do you wish you had loved someone else?'

'No, Mary. Even if you die tomorrow I will never regret what we have shared. We have known more love in a short time than most couples ever know. Of course I don't regret loving you. Don't ever say that again.'

We hold each other for a long time, feeling the warmth of closeness and being together. Then we kiss each other's tears away.

'Whatever happens, Richard, I want to know the truth. Don't hide anything from me. Promise?'

'I promise.'

'We need to make the most of the time we have left.'

'I know and we will.'

'Richard, do you think I am going to die of this illness?'

'Yes I do.'

'When? How long?'

'I don't know.'

'Do you think maybe God will heal me?'

Richard looks at me and sighs heavily. 'I don't know, Mary. I just don't know. Right now, I just feel angry with God.'

'But it's all we have to hold on to. We must hold on to hope. We must ...'

The day continues. It seems strange, the 'normality' of going about our daily affairs. It is time to collect Adam from school and Bethany from childcare. We go to the supermarket and buy pizzas for supper. We go home and bath the children. The routine remains unchanged. All the time Adam chatters about his day and we laugh at the funny stories he tells. Bethany toddles around after him. When they are safely tucked up in bed, Richard and I sit down and resume our conversation.

'I wish I knew more about the prognosis,' I say. 'I feel so powerless and helpless not knowing.'

'I could do a literature search on the computer.'

'Yes, and I could ring Mr Peach and Dr Gupta tomorrow.'

'Who shall we tell? We will need to tell family at some point.'

'I know, but not yet. I can't bear to think of all the sorrow it will bring. It will open so many wounds for Mum and Dad. Let's find out first what it means.'

I need to tell someone at church. The Elders met with me last Tuesday to pray for healing before I went to see Dr Smith. I had not been to an Elders' meeting before but, when I got the phone call to go back to clinic, I panicked and rang Ellie and told her what was happening.

'Okay,' she said. 'We need prayer support for you.' Ellie is really very sensible and practical about matters such as these. Being a nurse, too, she knew the implications.

In Rhiwbina Baptist Church there are six Elders, all experienced Christian men. David is our senior pastor who works full-time at the church and all the other Elders are part-time and have secular jobs. Each Elder takes on a certain area of responsibility and David oversees them all.

'We need to go and see them,' Ellie advised.

'Why? Can't we just pray ourselves? Isn't it a bit over the top going to an Elders' meeting?'

'Mary, I feel strongly that this situation is so serious that we need to have their wisdom in it. In the Bible it says that we should go and ask the Elders for prayer and anointing if we are sick.'

'Where does it say that?' Ellie has been to Bible College and knows a lot about scripture.

'In the book of James we read that if we are sick we should go to the Elders, be prayed for and be anointed with oil. The prayer offered in faith, it says, will be heard.'

'Why the oil, then?'

'The oil symbolizes God's blessing, that's all.'

So we went and the Elders prayed that the news would be good and that I would be strong enough to cope with the results.

'Ellie,' I say as I ring her now, 'it didn't work. The tumour is malignant. It's a met.'

'Okay, I'm coming over,' she says, and ten minutes later we are sitting together and I am crying again.

'Ellie, I think I've been through enough. Why is my cancer back now? What have I done wrong this time?'

'I'm not having any of that guilt stuff!' says Ellie. 'You have not caused the cancer. We live in a polluted, damaged world stuffed full of carcinogens. It's bad luck that you ended up with cancer but it's not your fault.'

'So I am not being punished?'

'No you are not! Listen – God loves you. His son Jesus died for you and bought you salvation. You're His child. Why would He punish you by giving you cancer?'

'Maybe I'm evil or something.'

'Maybe you were just in the wrong place at the wrong time. You are not evil. You're saved – how can you be evil?'

'Well, I'm hacked off with God. Why me? He always picks on me. I'm really angry at Him. He could have prevented me from getting sick again. But oh no! He just sits there in heaven and turns a blind eye.'

'Well, it's okay to be angry. God's big enough to take it.'

'Yes, well, He isn't big enough to take it away, is He? I'm sick of God, I'm going to give up on Him. I've had enough. I really have.'

'Hey, where is your faith? Come on, you told me a few weeks ago that if you weren't healed then you knew there was something better.'

'That was before … before I knew I was dying.' I feel a rising surge of anger against God, the doctors, the universe – everything. Anger, hot and boiling, as I think of my children, my husband, my life. 'It's not fair!' I yell. 'It's not bloody well fair!' I collapse in tears on the sofa and thump the cushions.

'Mary, you are angry. And that is normal. If you weren't angry I would be more worried.'

'So what am I going to do?'

'We take one day at a time. We find out the information. We pray and we get others to pray. We sort out the practical and go from there.'

'I don't want treatment. I can't bear the thought of chemo again.'

'Let's cross that bridge if we need to and not before.'

Two days later I receive a phone call from Velindre Hospital. I have an appointment to see an oncologist, Dr Saran, the following day.

Richard and I arrive early. It is a beautiful sunny day. The area is familiar, as Velindre is next to Whitchurch Hospital where I work. We have Bethany with us and her innocent joy takes away some of the desperate sadness we are feeling. Richard and I, holding hands tightly, are met with curious stares as we enter the outpatients' department looking young and healthy with our ridiculously small daughter. I see a glance of pity from the receptionist so I return a bright cheerful smile. I do not want pity. Richard and Bethany go in search of drinks and I sit in the waiting area, casting my eyes over the patients surrounding me.

The lady opposite me looks about forty. Her head is completely bald. I see the tight bandage compressing her arm and notice the slight asymmetry of her jumper. With my doctor's mind I diagnose her – breast cancer, lymph nodes taken out, had chemotherapy. She looks up at me and smiles a sorrowful, weary smile …

Another lady is bald. In fact, lots of the ladies are bald and, from time to time, they take off their wigs to brush them or scratch their heads. I wondered what it would look like and now I know.

I am brought back to the present by Bethany's return. She climbs all over me, restless and bored.

'I'll take her for a walk round,' I tell Richard and we set off to explore the corridor. Velindre is much more modern than Christie's was in 1983, but I recognize the signs and notices of a cancer hospital – CT scan, isotope department, radiotherapy treatment area. I feel depressed and older than my years. I walk past a door and spot the yellow radiation warning sign. I draw my breath in sharply. I saw it somewhere a long time ago. Not in Christie's, but way before. Where? Where did I see it? I look down at Bethany and she bends to pick something up.

'Bethany, don't pick that up – it's dirty, put it down, sweetheart …'

The tunnel was dark. We could hardly see but I was with my big brother, Martin, so I would be okay. The weekend was boring for children. All the grown-ups just sat around talking and laughing about things I didn't understand. So we went out to play and they let me come too. We went down an old disused mine. My brother and me got lost in a cave. I was frightened but my brother laughed at me and called me a scaredy-cat. I was not a scaredy-cat. I was seven and a big girl. After a while our eyes got used to the dark and we looked around to see what we could find. There was something in the corner – a big pile of black poles. They had all got yellow patterns on them and yellow is my favourite colour. And also the pattern was triangular and that is my favourite shape, so I thought I would look at them. I picked one up. It was very heavy and felt very cold as I dragged it over to show my big brother. I rested it on my knees and tried to pick it up again to impress Martin but he didn't seem impressed. He was cross. 'Put it down, Mary. Somebody found a bomb here once and stuff left over from wars and things.' I dropped the pole and it made a loud noise and rolled away. It was so pretty. I wish I could have taken it home …

I look at the sign on the door. 'Isotopes room – Danger! Radiation hazard.' Underneath the words I see the yellow triangles. I unlock the door to my subconscious mind. Perhaps I now know why the Limpet struck. Maybe it was, as Ellie said, the result of a polluted world and being in the wrong place at the wrong time. I am flooded with an incredible sense of relief and, at last, understanding.

I return to my seat in the waiting room. I shall tell my story to Richard later. It is too big to waste. The minutes pass and I feel more and more nervous. I have brought a book with me and try to read it but cannot concentrate. I flick instead through ancient copies of *Hello!* and look mindlessly at pictures of pop stars and glamorous women, pretending to myself that I am anywhere apart from this cancer hospital.

The nurse calls me over to be weighed. As I make my way to her office, I pass a trolley identical to the one I lay on all those years ago. A man is lying on it. His bones almost protrude through his stretched and waxy skin. He has a deep jaundice, his skin a golden brown and his eyes bright yellow. An oxygen mask covers his face and he is sleeping the sleep of exhaustion. He is being transferred out of Velindre Hospital. He is dying. I look at him and think: 'That will be me soon.' Thin, wasted, or, as we doctors would say, cachectic. I don't like the word; it is harsh and cruel. I do not want to look like that. I want to die beautiful and sparkly. I want to die with my make-up on and my hair in place. I want to wear my earrings and my nail polish and a gorgeous silk dress. I do not want to be a skeleton. I refuse.

Dr Saran tells me he is an oncologist specializing in childhood cancers and, because my tumour is a secondary which has spread from the original bone cancer, he will be looking after my care.

'I don't want you to keep anything from me,' I tell him. 'I have two young children and I really need to be able to plan for them.' I sound remarkably calm but inside I am not. I am trying to deal with myself in a detached, doctor way. It is the only way I can handle it.

'I understand and you will be able to read your notes. Ask as many questions as you like.'

'Is there any treatment for this secondary?'

'Well, the best thing has already been done – it has been removed. That is the first hurdle over. If this turns out to be the only secondary then surgery alone gives you a reasonable chance of staying well for some time.'

'So what is my prognosis?'

'We don't know.'

'Why don't you know?'

'This tumour has relapsed so late. There has never been a relapse recorded so late. As far as I know, the latest occurred at seven years after the original illness. We are dealing with an unknown beast here. We have to consider that it will not behave as other tumours do.'

'What if I have chemotherapy? Will that make a difference?'

'Again, we cannot say. It might help, but then it might not. I'm sorry to be vague but, as I said, this has never happened before. We cannot base your treatment on the results of a trial or previous experience because there aren't any.'

'If I had chemotherapy, what regime would I need? Or can't you tell that either?'

'Logically, we would have to use the same drugs as for a primary bone tumour. You have already had a previous course of Methotrexate, so we would have to go for an old-fashioned treatment because we can't use the same stuff twice.'

'And that would be?'

'I have to warn you, Mary,' says Dr Saran, cautiously, 'this regime of chemo would be very aggressive, very unpleasant and would carry a high risk of major side-effects. We would never use it as first-line treatment.'

'Okay, I understand. What does it involve?'

'The regime is called VIPA.'

I recognize the abbreviations of the drug names but I guess the treatment is also appropriately named after the venomous snake.

'So that would be Vincristine, Ifosfamide, Cisplatin and Adriamycin?'

'Correct.'

I look at Richard in horror.

'Vincristine could cause bone marrow failure and nerve toxicity?'

'Yes, it's a possibility.'

'Ifosfamide … stomach problems and nausea … Cisplatin would cause total hair loss and, possibly, bone marrow problems and kidney failure?'

186

'Yes, it is possible.'

'And Adriamycin is the biggie – that could cause heart failure.'

'Yes. As I said, it is a very toxic regime.'

'How toxic? Give me some figures.'

'A death rate of five per cent and a fifteen per cent risk of major side-effects. The unpleasant minor side-effects go without saying. We have excellent links with the intensive care unit at University Hospital if these should occur.'

'Yes, so do I. My husband works as the clinical fellow there,' I say quickly.

Richard and Dr Saran look at me warily as I laugh emptily at my black joke.

'Would I become menopausal?' I continue.

'Almost certainly.'

'It would be hell, right? Six months of my life would be unbearable and then six months more to recover from it?'

'Yes, I would agree with your assessment.' Dr Saran looks at me apologetically.

'If it was you – would you have it?'

'I have to offer it to you. I have to give you the option.'

'But would you have it? Would you go through with it if you were me?' I ask impatiently. I want to be told straight.

'No, I wouldn't.'

'Thank you for being honest. I don't want it either. The risks are too high. I would lose a year of my life for no certain benefit and I would go through immense suffering. I need to spend time with the children and I wouldn't be able to do that if I had VIPA.'

'Okay. You need to be sure, though, that if it does spread you feel you did everything you could.'

'I know. I will think about it some more, but we have looked all through the current literature and talked to my previous specialists and the studies seem to back up the decision that I – we – have made.'

I look at Richard.

'I wouldn't go through that,' he says. 'And I certainly can't watch you go through it. But I just want to be clear. If Mary did have that treatment, would it guarantee a cure or just improve her chances of remaining clear?'

'We are definitely not talking cure. It might improve her chances but we really don't know for sure.'

'I think we are both agreed,' I say. 'We cannot go through that or allow the children to go through watching it, either. If surgery is the most important aspect of treatment, then we will stick with that.'

Dr Saran pauses and then continues. 'The next fact we have to be sure of is whether you have any further spread of the cancer.'

'But I had tests before my surgery. I thought the rest of my body was clear?'

'It's a couple of months now since you had those tests. I think we should repeat them and look more closely at the rest of your body. We know we are dealing with a very unusual tumour here. We can't be too careful.'

'So what tests do I need?'

'A whole-body CT scan and an isotope bone scan. That should be sufficient. We need to check out your brain, bones, liver, lungs and lymph nodes.'

'Yes,' I sigh. 'I know, I know. I've done it before. Just go ahead and book them ...'

This test was the most important, I was told – the isotope one. If there were any bad bits in the bone, they would glow brightly. I had two of these scans at the Victoria before but now I had to have this one at Christie's, too. As the porter tucked me into my wheelchair, Vera came up to me. There is a young man, Martin, here to visit you, she said. Oh, it will be my brother ... he can come with me to my scan. Then I saw him walking down the ward and it was Martyn – my ex. Mary, he said, I really needed to visit you. That's nice, I said, but I'm okay. Do you mind if I come with you to your test? No. But it will be boring. So he walked beside the wheelchair while I puzzled over why he had come to see me. Manchester is a long way from Blackpool. It was a weekday so he must have skived off school. I felt quite proud he had made so much effort. While I had the test, Martyn took hold of my hand, can you believe it? He didn't say anything, he just carried on stroking my hand. I drifted off to sleep and when I woke up he looked at me and smiled and asked me if I was all right. I almost thought maybe he loved me, but why would he love me now when I have no leg and my hair is about to fall out? He looked at the screen. I can't see any blobs, he said. Me neither, I said. It's probably clear then, I told him. But he looked so sad, so we talked about school instead and he made me laugh. Then he came back to the ward and Vera drew the curtains around us. I sort of wanted to talk about him and me but then I was not sure what to say. Mary, you know I did care about you, he said. He looked at me for a long, long time and I felt a bit embarrassed. There was a pain in Martyn's eyes that I had not seen before. I knew what it was, for I too felt the same – it was guilt. That is how it makes you feel, cancer. Guilty. As he walked away down the ward I suddenly realized why he had come and why he looked at me so strangely. He thinks I'm going to die …

It is now a month since Dr Smith gave me the shocking news. We are in June 1999. I feel quite optimistic again today. The cancer is back and it has spread to my lung but now it has been removed my outlook might be quite good. Nothing is guaranteed, of course, but if I get through these tests then I can get on with recovering.

I ring Dr Gupta again and seek his reassurance. 'Well, Mary,' he says, 'I know it is a big worry for you, but our experience is that when a single met is taken out at thoracotomy the results are good. We would see it as a curative procedure and we wouldn't give chemotherapy, either.'

'So it's not a death sentence then?'

'No – as long as it is the only place it has spread to. Do you have any symptoms anywhere, any pain or anything you cannot explain?'

'No, no – well, only the usual gynae aches and pains.'

I sit in the garden and try to relax and read my Bible. I've been trying to pray and read the Psalms every day – holding on to God is the only way I can cope with all this. I find it difficult to concentrate but the Psalms are easy to read and seem to speak to me in my current situation. As I am reading, I think about the conversation with Dr Gupta: '… the usual gynae aches and pains …'

I still have that nagging pain in my pelvis. In fact, recently it has been pretty severe. I start to worry about it now. Maybe it is my lymph nodes at the top of my Little Leg. Perhaps it's spread there, too. I ring Nigel, the consultant who did the ultrasound scans. Maybe he will be able to reassure me.

'Nigel – it's Mary Self.'

'Hiya, Heartsink! Please don't tell me you're having another baby!'

'No, I wish it was that simple. I haven't been well. I had a tumour taken out of my lung – it was a secondary from my bone cancer.'

There is a long silence.

'Mary, I'm really sorry. That's very unusual – I thought it was all ancient history now.'

'Well, it was. I had basically stopped worrying about it. The cancer specialists are all astonished – it's never been recorded for a bone tumour to relapse this late on.'

'Is there anything I can do?'

'Well, I did have a question. Do you remember the pain I had in my pelvis? Well, I still have it. I was kind of worrying that it might be something … maybe my lymph nodes.'

There is another, much longer silence.

'I was wondering – would lymph nodes have shown up when we did the scans?'

'No, the scan would not have picked up lymph nodes.'

We chat about the operation and I fill him in on my daughter's progress.

'I wanted to thank you, Nigel,' I say suddenly.

'What for?'

'For all that you did when I was having Bethany and after losing the baby. I couldn't have got through it without you.'

'Yes, you could – but it's nice of you to say so. Let me know how the tests go, won't you?'

I put the phone down with a sinking feeling. Nigel sounded worried, too.

I decide to tell my family about the Penny. I cannot keep it from them any longer.

I sit on the stairs while Richard speaks to my dad. I listen to him being very calm and practical. It is not how I feel – not how Richard feels. He hands the phone to me. My dad's voice is full of loving concern. I can tell he is fighting back tears. I listen to him but I don't hear, I am too full of confusion. I feel a burden of sorrow that once again they are going through so much pain. The familiar guilt creeps in.

My brothers call me, sounding awkward. They tell me they love me and that is all that matters. Then my sisters call.

'We are here for you,' they say. 'We are behind you and we are with you in spirit.' But I hear the sadness in their voices. Sisters three, we say, and it needs to stay three. I put down the phone and look at Richard. We are sitting on the stairs together. I wrap my arms around him and cry. I want to be enfolded in love. I want to be held in warmth. Nothing matters apart from our love, our life and the good times we have shared.

'Oh Richard,' I say to him, 'what shall we do? I can't bear leaving you.'

Our tears mingle with kisses in our despair.

The following day I attend for my CT scan. My friend Ceri, a Christian from Rhiwbina Baptist Church, comes with me. She has received treatment for breast cancer at this hospital. I feel an easy camaraderie. I do not need to explain the uncertainty to her.

'Ceri,' I ask her. 'Do you think I'm in denial? I feel this peace inside me. Almost as if I'm especially close to God at the moment.'

'No, I don't think you're in denial,' she says in her matter-of-fact way. 'I think you know that even though this is tough, really tough, you can do this in God's strength.'

'But I feel I also need to be real. I remember, first time around, I used to think I had to have a big cheesy grin on my face, saying the right words and looking holy.'

'Well, Jesus was human, too. He had real human emotions. He got angry, in the temple, and He knew despair in the garden of Gethsemane. I think He understands all the emotions you are going through.'

I smile at her. I know she is right. Anger and sadness are perfectly reasonable emotions to experience. I don't have to pretend.

The second test, the isotope bone scan, is the following day and Ceri again accompanies me. I lie on the couch after receiving the injection and strain my neck to see the screen. Ceri holds my hand throughout and reads aloud from the scriptures. The scanner moves down my body and small green dots, depicting my bones, appear on screen. I can see my bladder glowing brightly where the isotopes have collected in my urine. The dots begin to form the outline of my pelvis. I notice a discrepancy. The left side is brighter than the right side.

I look away for a few minutes. I think back to the three times that I waited for my pregnancy tests to develop. How badly I wanted to see a bright dot then. Now I close my eyes and pray. 'Please, God, I don't want any blobs.' After maybe five minutes, I look again. It is there, glowing – a bright green blob. I look away and wait. Maybe the left side has cooked before the right. After another ten minutes I look again and my heart sinks. The despair hits me like a tidal wave. There is the blob – a horrible glowing blob. It is a hot-spot. I know it should not be there. I have the same feelings of resentment I had when I first saw the Limpet and the Penny. It is a Blob in my body in the wrong place. You are an invader, an alien, possessing me and destroying me. Go away, Blob. Go away! Spreading secretively and flowing out into my bones. Sending down your greedy tentacles to devour my health and strip away my life.

191

I will not allow you to kill me, to suck me dry. You are, as you have always been, illegitimate. You are, and you will always be, a bastard.

'He will give His angels charge over you,' reads Ceri from Psalm 91.

'Lest you hurt your foot against a stone.' I finish.

You will not destroy me – Limpet, Penny, Blob. You will not.

A week later I go to see Dr Saran and discuss the results of my CT and isotope tests. It is now almost halfway through June; time is moving on. I have not spoken of the Blob to anybody. Maybe I was wrong. Maybe it is just one of those normal variations. I wait anxiously with Richard, passing time by flicking through the pages of yet another ancient copy of *Hello!* Last night I went to see the Elders again. They prayed over me for healing once more and they anointed me with oil, too. As they did so, I prayed inside my mind desperately for totally clear tests. I asked God to take away the Blob. I heard Him answer: 'Trust Me, Mary, trust Me even unto death.' It was not what I wanted to hear. I wanted something like 'I am the God who heals you.' So I got terrified. Is it wrong to want healing before anything else? I know I should want to be with Jesus so much that it should seem much better than being here on earth. But, in all honesty, what I really want, deep down, is to see my kids grow up and to wake up every morning in the same bed as Richard. Is that wrong?

Dr Saran is sitting with a nurse – a Macmillan nurse. Why is she here? She was not here last time. I look at her angrily. I do not want her here. I know what they do. They are palliative care nurses whose job is to relieve symptoms. My mouth is dry and I feel sick. Dr Saran has my bone scan pictures and my CT scan pinned up on the light box.

'Mary, we have been looking at your results,' he says calmly, in a voice that is too kind.

'What do they show?'

'There is a problem.'

'What kind of problem?'

'This. See, just here. That is your pelvic bone, left side. Do you have any symptoms there?'

'Yes. Pain.'

'Show me.'

I point to the area.

'Has it got worse recently?'

'Yes, it has.'

'Mary, you know what this is, don't you?'

192

'It's a met, right?'

'I'm afraid that's what we all think.'

I sit and stare at the Blob, hating it. Strange how different it is from the Limpet and the Penny. It is insidious and creeping. The silence in the room is heavy and oppressive. The nurse reaches out for my hand but I take it away. I don't want anybody to acknowledge my enemy. It is not there, not really. If I close my eyes and open them again, it will be gone, I know. I try, but the first thing I see is the Blob. Blob the bastard.

'So how can you treat it, then?' I say brightly, smiling incongruously at Dr Saran. 'What do I need this time? Can you operate?'

'No, it is in the most difficult of places. It is at the base of your spine.'

'How about chemo?'

'We could give you VIPA …'

I interrupt quickly. 'Great, do it. When shall we start?'

'However, I must stress that it would only buy you time.'

'How much time?'

'We don't know – maybe none.'

'Okay, so I'll have radiotherapy.'

'Mary, this type of problem doesn't respond to radiotherapy.'

'So where does that leave me?'

Dr Saran looks at me and then the nurse and my life begins to slow down.

'What are you telling me? What are you trying to say?'

There is another silence and I need to fill it. My voice is loud now and insistent with the anger of it all. Are you telling me I'm going to die? Is that what you're telling me? Don't tell me that. I'm thirty-four. You must have made a mistake. The nurse reaches over and touches me and I shake her off. Go away go away all of you just get out of here leave me alone and I'm crying crying I am filled with an anger so big and so real. Just go away I'm not dying I'm not I'm fine so just go and leave me alone. I stand up and push them out of the room and I'm yelling just go away. Mary, says the doctor. Don't you understand me? Just get out. Richard speaks I can't hear him. Something leave her here it's what she wants. I'll talk to you. Go way I am shouting. Who at? Is it the doctor is it the Limpet is it the Penny is it the Blob or is it death now staring me in the face when I don't know how I don't know why why why I don't know oh God I don't know and they are gone. I am crying crying crying for Richard for my children for all that will be taken away please please don't take me away from them. Tears are hot and flow down my face and pool on to my hands and I sob loudly and angrily.

My God, my God, why have You forsaken me, I whisper, and in the room there is a Presence and I know he is there again the same Presence eight foot tall and bright. I am enfolded in his peace and held close and safe and warm and loving just like a mother comforting a baby I am soothed and I whimper as I rest my head on the couch next to me. I don't know where the Presence is, he is all around and yet he is somewhere. My heart stills now and my breathing slows and I feel as if I am curled up in a giant hand, safe in the Father's hand, it is like a gentle breeze blowing through my soul and calming me, calming me, my child don't be scared, don't be scared. I sit up and my eyes feel cooler, my mind clearer. I can do it, I know I can do it. I am dying. I can die. I know how to die. The Presence will lead me. Through ... the unknown. Through ...

'I'm sorry,' I say as I walk back into Dr Saran's consulting room.

'That's okay. Anger is normal in these circumstances.'

'I am going to die of this illness, aren't I?'

'Yes. I'm afraid that is what it looks like.'

'When? Can you tell me when?'

'It's impossible to say. We can never give an exact timescale. We really don't know. But I don't think it will be in the next few months.'

Silence.

Disbelief.

'I think I would like to go now.'

'All right. You need time to think. Let's meet again next week.'

We leave his office. It seems almost as if all the other patients know as I walk out. I feel strangely transparent, as if everybody I pass is able to see 'Hello, I'm dying' written on my face. I feel embarrassed and awkward and shy, as if my new state of being incurable is obvious to all.

'Where shall we go?' I ask Richard. We look at each other, numb with shock. 'Shall we go somewhere nice?'

'I suppose so. I don't really know.'

'I guess we still need to eat. I can't think straight.'

'Me neither.'

We take each other's hands and stand in the hospital entrance.

'It isn't true is it? Tell me it isn't true,' I implore Richard. I feel as if I am in a fog. I do not want it to be true and neither does Richard. 'Let's pretend it isn't true,' I say brightly. 'Come on, let's go for a wonderful meal. Let's go to that lovely country restaurant that we go to for special treats.'

It is a beautiful sunny day and we sit on a bench in a scented garden. 'The lambs are quite big now,' I say. 'It's June already. I feel as if I have missed the spring. I can't remember seeing the lambs when they were tiny.' I gaze at the scene before me. The rolling Welsh hills and the fresh green valleys. 'We must make the most of the summer,' I say, sadly. Suddenly life has shortened to seasons instead of years.

Richard grabs me round the waist and puts his head in my lap. 'Oh Mary – I can't bear the thought of losing you.' I bury my head in his hair and recognize the familiar smell of my best friend and lover. It is strange how primitive I feel. It is as if I know every atom of my husband. I cannot bear the thought of leaving. We cling to each other, weeping softly together, like drowning children holding on to half of our lives.

'Have I ever told you, Mary,' whispers Richard, 'how much I love you?'

'Many times, but say it again.' We kiss and it is the most beautiful kiss I shall ever know. Touch, smell, taste, exquisitely combined in a love heightened magnificently by the shadow of death.

Later on we gather with the children in our back garden. I watch my two miracles playing in the evening sunshine. Adam is throwing a ball for Bethany to run after. She laughs with joy, her head thrown back and her teeth gleaming white, her mischievous smile captured for ever in my memory. Adam comes and sits on my lap in his tired, affectionate way.

'I love you, Mum,' he says, and nestles close to my heart. I stroke his hair and kiss his tousled head.

'I love you too, Adam.'

He hugs me tightly. 'Best mummy in the world!' he laughs and scampers off again to play in youthful and blissful innocence …

How long until I die, I think to myself. I haven't even begun to live my life. I am only a child. I have not done anything, seen anything, lived anything yet.

'If You take me from them, Lord,' I pray silently, 'give them a mother figure. I cannot bear the thought of them being alone …'

'Ellie – I need to talk to you. The bone scan showed another met. It's called the Blob.'

'Okay,' she says calmly. 'Well, I guess we need to talk things through. I will tell the Elders and we'll get them praying. Do you feel angry?'

'I did at first but it passed quite quickly. Now I just keep thinking about time and how much of it I might have.'

Time, time that uncertain commodity. It is time I crave. I am so young, so young. I didn't know seventeen-year-olds could die of cancer.

'If I could only see the children grow up a little. Bethany is so young. She won't …' My voice cracks and I sob into the phone.

'I know,' Ellie says after a while. 'I know.'

'One day at a time then?' I ask, once I have controlled myself.

'Yes, one day at a time. Let's just get you through one day at a time.'

'I need to see Nigel,' I say to his secretary later in the day. 'It's really urgent.'

'Come up tomorrow,' she says.

I am not sure why I feel he can help me. I suppose it is because he saved my life once, and the life of my daughter. I need to gather my support around me now. I cannot lean on my family, for they will need support too. We all have to live under the shadow of this diagnosis.

I see now that we all have cancer one way or another.

'Hiya, Heartsink,' Nigel greets me. 'How did the tests go, are they clear?'

'No, I'm afraid not.'

He looks at me tentatively. I'm not sure how to tell him or why it is so difficult.

'The pain in my pelvis – it's a secondary in my bone.'

Nigel sits upright quickly. 'Oh Mary, I'm so sorry. Can they remove it? Or give you treatment?'

I shake my head and look at my hands. This is the first time I have told anybody, apart from Richard and Ellie. I am determined not to cry.

'It's going to kill me, Nigel.' A tear plops on to my hand and I brush it away. He is stunned, in silence. He looks at me. 'Oh God. Oh my God.' There are tears in his eyes too, now. We sit for a few minutes. I know what he will say. He puts his head in his hands and then looks up at me.

196

'Should we have done more, Mary? Do you think we should have done more?'

There was a pain in Martyn's eyes that I had not seen before. I knew what it was, for I too felt the same – it was guilt. That is how it makes you feel, cancer. Guilt …

'No, Nigel, honestly I don't. I hadn't thought about my cancer for years. It was over and done with. I was worried about developing a new type of cancer, maybe in my ovaries, because I knew they were at risk, but a secondary – I just didn't think it was possible now.'

'Should we have done a CT scan after Bethany was born?'

'Well, even if we had, it would still have been the same outcome, bone mets are invariably fatal. I guess I've just had one year less of worrying about it.'

Nigel seems to sink back in his chair and, although he looks sad, I know I have released him from any guilt he may have felt. I wish it could be as simple for me.

'You're being horribly brave, Mary,' Nigel says, and I smile.

'It's weird, Nigel. All the time when I was worrying about the cancer coming back, last year, it seemed as if it was the worst thing I could ever face. When I had to face it … well, somehow it wasn't as fearsome as I thought. I mean, it's awful, don't get me wrong, but in some ways I feel strangely at peace now. Almost as if I don't have to fight any more.'

'So what can I do to help? Anything?'

'Well, I guess you could just be there as a good friend – I need to enjoy life for the next … the next … however long.'

'Count me in on the parties, then.' We laugh and hug. His hug is comforting and strong and I draw something from him.

'Actually,' I say, 'you make me feel brave.'

'Mary, you are brave. I know you are. I've seen you face so much already.'

'I am scared though – a little.'

'I know you are. I would be scared a lot.'

'I'm not scared of being dead because I know I will be with God in heaven. I'm scared of the getting there.'

'Hey, don't think like that. We will all make sure you get the best care – all your medical friends. I promise.'

'Thanks, Nigel.'

197

'Be brave.'

'I will. I promise.'

I do not feel very brave as I walk away from his office but I feel comforted knowing that I have my medical friends to help me. I begin to construct in my head a way of getting through this vale of death. I sit outside on a bench overlooking a fountain in the hospital grounds. I pray …

I am walking through a wooded valley. The cliffs each side tower above me. At the end I see the most beautiful glade, all shady and green and cool. There is a path winding into the distance. I don't know how long it is or what awaits in the parts I can't see. Beside the path there are hundreds of scented, colourful plants and butterflies dancing amid the blooms. It looks really pretty as long as I don't look too far to either side – where there are brambles and nettles and potholes and maybe fierce animals lurking near rocks and caves. But it's all right as long as I keep my eyes fixed on the glade. The sun sparkles through the canopy of leaves. Above the beautiful clearing at the end of the valley there is a pair of enormous hands. They are the hands of a man, strong and capable. They are the hands of a worker and a healer. They are scarred but beautiful. In the hands I place my entire family. They are held in complete love. Richard is holding Bethany in his arms and Adam holds his dad's hand. I place my two sisters at either side of Richard. They are mother figures. Then I place my mum and dad right over the scars on the enormous hands so they will be especially safe. My two brothers are at either side of my sisters. I cannot see the rest of our family but I know they are there in the hands too. Instead of walking away from them I am walking towards them. A huge waterfall is cascading down from the enormous hands and the water is crystal clear. I can feel the spray as I walk through the beautiful wood. I think the butterflies are maybe prayers because I notice they are all flying towards the enormous hands and sometimes they settle there and then disappear into the scars. I am only wearing a thin t-shirt and my feet are bare. I cannot walk this path like that, I think, but in front of me I see some armour. First I don my belt of truth, made of creaky leather with a shiny buckle. Then I put on my breastplate to cover and protect my heart. That is righteousness. Next, my shoes which are really like big boots with sturdy soles and big thick laces. They are the gospel of peace. Then I pick up my beautiful, ornate golden shield. It's not heavy at all. In fact it does not weigh anything. Faith. I place my golden helmet over my head to protect my thoughts. Salvation. Then I take up my huge sword, gleaming, sharp and keen. The Spirit. Now I am ready. All I need is a group of trusted friends to keep me company and help me continue walking when I get tired or despondent. Ellie is there already. She is Kindness. Next I put Nigel, and he is Courage. Ellie holds one hand and Nigel walks beside me. Off we all go towards the beautiful glade and the enormous hands. I think God has shown me a way through dying.

The journey has only begun, I think, so I will invite others along the way. I choose my fellow travellers carefully. There is no time to waste. I cannot afford to get it wrong. Do not pity me. Help me. Stand with me. Be my friend. Cry when I cry. Laugh when I laugh. Celebrate my life with me. Be there. I know I will not escape death but I do not want to be attacked by the evil Despair or the fearsome Pain. I want to get to the enormous hands without too many horrors.

Towards the end of June, I contact my friend Sue, a consultant anaesthetist in Swansea. We sit in a lovely restaurant, order a delicious meal and some fine champagne and I tell her my plan.

'What I need is a group of friends who will stick with me. Kind of a support group. I want to be happy and have some good times. I want to be able to talk openly about my fears and worries. I want strong people who will not baulk if I mention the Death word.'

'Well, it sounds like a really positive approach,' she says, as if it is the sort of thing we talk about every day. 'Let's call your support group the Band of Merry Men and Women.'

'I want people who can help me make medical decisions too – so doctors are better. I really don't need tea or sympathy. I need practical help and I need openness.'

'Okay, so who have you in mind? We don't want any miserable folk, do we?'

'Absolutely not. Everybody involved has to have the feel-good factor.'

'As opposed to the feel-bad factor?'

'You've got it. Now I want you to head up the group. Do you mind?'

'No, but why me?'

'You've always been so accepting of everything I have been through. So you stand for …'

'Permission?'

'That's it! Permission to do and say whatever is needed. I thought of Dafydd, too.'

Sue nods wisely. Dafydd is her colleague.

'I'm going to have to make a lot of very difficult decisions about my care, especially areas such as pain control. And I am so scared of the pain. Dafydd has always been the sort of doctor I aspired to be. He is knowledgeable, compassionate and sensible. He also has loads of contacts.'

'Great choice. So what does he stand for?'

'Skill. He stands for Skill.'

'Anybody else?'

'Mark in Cardiff. Another doctor. He runs marathons and he stands for Endurance.'

'Okay. Carry on.' She writes down everything in a little notebook I have brought with me.

'Tim, my friend, is Laughter. Cathy, my psychiatrist friend, is Compassion. Valerie is Calm. And David – my friend in Australia – is Sensitivity. Alison and Brian in Swansea are Wisdom.'

'No family?'

'No, because the whole point is to protect my family so I can enjoy being with them. I don't want to spoil our times by burdening them.'

Our meals arrive and we soon drink the bottle of champagne. 'Let's order another,' says Sue. 'After all, you only die once.' Soon we are gloriously and happily tipsy and we laugh until our sides ache.

'Okay, so is there anything you want to do over the next few months? I mean, do you have any unfulfilled ambitions?'

'I'm sure I do. Let me think.'

Sue turns to a clean page in the notebook. 'They can be as outrageous as you want.'

'Okay, how's this for starters? I've never worn a G-string and I've always wanted one!'

I have never eaten garlic bread before.

Sue talks out loud as she writes down 'black, lacy G-string'. Two men at the table behind us stare and we both explode into fits of laughter. 'I'll buy you that, then,' adds Sue. 'What else?'

'I've never been to Amsterdam.'

I've never been abroad.

'Naughtiness in Amsterdam,' Sue mutters.

'A romantic weekend in Paris.'

I've never made love with anybody and I'll never wear a beautiful white wedding dress.

'Great. Absolutely great so far. You're going to be busy.'
    'I've never been to a live rugby match or seen a big-name rock band on stage.'

I've never drunk red wine in a grown-up restaurant.

'Rugby international … rock band.'
    'I want to see all of Shakespeare's plays.'

I haven't even seen medical school. I might not even make it to my A levels.

'Anything else?'
    'I want to take Adam and show him his birthplace in Oz and snorkel the Barrier Reef.'

And, do you know, I have never even held a sweet, newborn baby. Let alone had my own child which will never, ever be. And that makes me so unhappy.

'Is that it?'
    'I might add New York at Christmas if I make it that far.'
    'All right,' says Sue, giggling at the list. 'I can't believe we're having this conversation.' She adds, 'You know, I think the Band of Merry Men and Women should have a theme tune, a feel-good anthem.'
    'Great idea! Something really upbeat, good dance number. Dancing always cheers me up.'
    'Any ideas?' she asks. We pause and think.
    'I've got it!' I answer. ' "Stayin' Alive" – the Bee Gees!'
    We collapse, helpless with laughter. The restaurant is about to close and the waiter comes over to clear our table.
    'You seem to have had a great time, ladies,' he says. 'What are you celebrating?'
    Sue and I look at each other and burst into laughter again.

201

'Mary is dying,' explains Sue. 'We are celebrating her life.'

'How can you be so brave and happy?' he asks.

'I guess I have hope because of my faith. Yes, that's it. I have Hope.'

There are many things to organize. First, I am in pain. The Blob is beginning to creep further into my bones and now it is hurting me a great deal. I contact Dafydd and we meet up one sunny day to talk about my pain control.

'I think we need to sort out a regime which you can manage yourself and increase when you need to,' suggests Dafydd.

'That sounds exactly what I would like, too.'

So we come up with a scale of painkillers, starting with the weaker ones and working up gradually. At the moment I am on medium-strength but soon I will be requiring stronger ones.

'Mary, have you thought about how your pain is going to be managed when it becomes more severe?'

'Well, no. I haven't felt able to think about it. I know that there is a palliative care team because they've told me about it at Velindre. I guess I don't feel ready for that yet.'

'Can you explain a little?'

'Well, once I start going along to see the hospice team, it's like admitting that I really am dying. I'm not quite at the point of admitting that yet.'

'Yes, I see – but what about when you need to start on morphine or something similar?'

'I suppose I want to avoid getting to that stage. I can't face the thought of needing to be on strong and addictive opiates for my pain. Then it really will feel as if I'm dying.'

'Well, just as long as you know that when that time comes we will all help you get through it.'

'I know, Dafydd. Truly, I know.'

I am getting worse. Slowly, gradually, the pain is becoming more severe. I am getting weaker, too. But as I grow physically weaker, in other ways I become so much stronger. The word is now out that I am dying. Many churches and Christians have begun to pray for my complete healing. We pray, too, as a family: Richard, myself and Adam. Every night we sit together and we each say a prayer.

Adam's is always the same: 'Please, Lord Jesus, make my mummy better. Amen.' Sometimes it makes me cry and sometimes it makes me smile. His faith is so young and simple and he never questions whether

202

it will happen. He just expects it. I worry sometimes that his faith will be destroyed when I die, but everybody tells me children are resilient.

When I pray I always hear the same words enter my head about trusting even unto death. I remember the survival vow sometimes and I try to say it to myself but it doesn't ring true any more. I know it is hard for others to understand, but I am okay about dying – I really am. It doesn't seem too bad at present. I just go around enjoying myself and trying to make the most of every day. I will probably take quite a long time to die at this rate. I have started to plan again in milestones – if I make it to Christmas, the millennium, things like that. I think it may even take a few years. My way of coping seems to be working – the prayers are being said and all my fellow travellers are right alongside me, helping me to walk the valley. I feel really close to the people I love. My friends confide more, too. Being a dying woman is a little like hearing confessions. I feel a bit like I imagine a priest does – I'll take the secrets with me to the grave. Perhaps, too, my friends feel I have this closeness to the other side. And I do feel like that.

It is almost like dwelling in God's heart. When I pray, it isn't just words any more. It is more like being with Him. I never, ever felt like this before. I read my Bible and I don't have to try to take the words in: it is like eating a nourishing meal – chew, swallow, grow. Every morsel seems particularly delicious, too. I don't feel mad at God about dying any more. I'll miss everybody and it breaks my heart sometimes, but the anger has gone. And I've stopped trying to talk God into things by bargaining. I suppose I feel an overwhelming sadness; but in that sadness there is also a kind of beautiful poignant peace. I am not struggling or fighting. I can accept now that I am dying. I want to be healed – I would like that so much. But if I don't get healed … well, that's okay, too.

As July arrives, I receive an e-mail from David, one of my medical friends from way back when I lived in Swansea. Now he lives in Australia and we send each other long and chatty mails. He is always optimistic and cheerful. I love to hear about his adventures from Down Under. I read his message with a sense of growing hope today.

'I think some people have this ability to overcome serious illness,' he shares. 'I could never believe in your God but I know how strong your faith is. You must not give up hope. Sometimes tumours regress even when they shouldn't. The impossible happens. There must be some side of life and death that we don't fully know about. If anybody can harness that, you can.'

'Thanks, David,' I reply. And then I add – because I have not seen him since carefree days living on the Welsh coast – 'If you don't make it back here and the worst happens, I want you to remember us sitting side by side on the beach. Remember the day we went for that long swim across Horton Bay and sat shivering in the evening sun? That's how I want you to remember me.'

I can do it, I think to myself. I can cope with this death business.

I am beginning to tick things off my ambitions list. I now have my black lacy G-string and believe me it looks great. However it is rather uncomfortable and personally I am not sure what all the fuss is about. I have also booked a holiday. Guess where? Australia! Richard and I are taking Adam to see his birthplace. I am so excited, and we have already contacted our friends over there. We are going for the whole of August and little Bethany is going to stay with her grandparents. This is our special trip with Adam. I am going to snorkel the Barrier Reef, too. When I return I am going to start doing the other things on my list.

But in the first week in July I feel so ill. My pain is awful. The moderately strong tablets aren't helping. I know the next step is morphine-type drugs. This morning I awoke to find strange things happening to my body. My asthma has started again and my eyes and fingers are all swollen like fat sausages. I keep sweating all over – I am drenched and soaking several times a day. I feel so weak I can hardly comb my hair, and I cannot even carry Bethany. My breasts are full of milk, too. It is all so weird. I know these symptoms are because of the Blob chucking histamine – spitting poison – into my body. I have seen it happen to my dying patients. It hurts so much. I don't know what to do.

'Nigel – something weird is going on.' I briefly tell him my symptoms.

'Come up and see me now,' he says, 'we need to get you sorted.'

I sit in his office and cry. 'I am thirty-four and I've got two kids and I'm dying. What am I going to do?' I am upset and sweating and hurting.

He takes both my hands in his and looks at me.

'You need to see your oncologist – today.'

'But I know what he will say. I'm not going.'

'Mary, you have to go. Please. You have to get help. Maybe the symptoms can be improved – certainly the pain can.'

'I don't want to hear the words.'

'Come on, you're brave, remember? Let's phone him and make an appointment.'

'Okay. I'll go.' I feel brave again now.

And so I go to see Dr Saran and it is terrible.

'It's spreading widely now, isn't it?'

'I'm afraid it is.'

'Do I do the things I want to do?'

'I think you should.'

Fear.

Loneliness.

Pain.

The mobile phone connects and I hear Courage.

'Hi, Mary. How did it go?'

'Terrible.'

'Where are you?'

'Sitting on the Wenallt Hill.'

'And what are you doing there?'

'Looking at the cemetery.'

There is a silence as Nigel takes this in.

'I have my Bible and I'm reading about miracles and feeling hacked off with God because I'm dying. Where are you?'

'On the train. Coming back from London. So why are you sitting looking at the cemetery? Are you picking your plot?'

I laugh. 'I suppose I am. I would really like one with a massive cherry tree. I love blossom. It always reminds me of when I knew I was expecting Bethany.'

'How do you feel?'

'Scared, Nigel. Is that okay?'

'Yes, that's okay.'

'It hurts, too. The Blob hurts me now so much.'

'Look, I think we need to talk about the palliative care team. Talk it through with Dafydd and come over tomorrow. I know just the person.'

So here I am sitting in the hospice clinic. I have to see Dr Jefferson. Nigel says she is a Christian. Dafydd thinks it is time to talk to her, too. It's weird. I feel even now, seventeen years on, the same childlike fear. I still have the need to hide away and protect my family from how I am feeling. I really don't want to cause them any more pain. I worry about saying to my Christian friends about the fear. Maybe I shouldn't be scared if I am a true believer. I mean, heaven isn't meant to be scary, is it? I am meant to believe in an after-life, and I do. What I am scared of is the getting there. I have seen so many people die. Some deaths are not very pleasant. Somebody at church said again the other day about

205

how they couldn't wait to be dead so they could be with Jesus. 'Fine,' I said, 'but what about the bit in between?' Is that doubt? I don't think so. I wonder how Jesus felt dragging up Calvary with the cross on His back. I bet He didn't think, 'I can't wait to be in heaven.' I bet He thought, 'How much will it hurt?' I bet He was scared like I am. In some ways I feel easier, telling Nigel and Sue and Dafydd I am scared, because they don't believe in God. There is no faith to damage.

When my friends visit me from school, I tell them it's okay. I tell them God is using me for His glory. I smile this big smile. I call it my plaster saint smile.

In a clinic waiting room everybody shares a bond. Here it is death. The lady next to me is quite old. Probably about seventy. She turns every so often to look at me. She is puzzled by my age. I ignore her for a while. I am not ready to talk and I can sense her curiosity building up. I hide my head in another copy of *Hello!* This is a really ancient one. I wonder gloomily how many people who have read this copy are now dead. Soon the lady can no longer keep silent.

'When did you get your cancer?' she asks.

'Seventeen years ago.'

'Oh. And it's only terminal now, then?'

'I found out a few weeks ago.'

'You are very young.'

State the obvious, why not, I feel like saying; but instead I reply: 'I'm thirty-four.' I stare at the magazine picture of Michael Jackson in the vague hope she will not ask the next, inevitable question, but she does.

'I see you're married. Do you have children?'

'Two. Seven and eighteen months.'

She draws her breath in sharply. 'That's awful, terrible. And I thought it was bad for me. Mine's in my brain now. Spread from my breast. Nothing they can do. But my kids are all grown up. In fact I have grand-children. I'll miss them.'

Now my heart is bursting. My eyes are holding back floods of tears. I feel so angry that my raw pain has been touched. It is my pain, I own it, I control it. Not a woman I have never met. She should know better, I think. She must know what it's like for me.

'Please,' I say to her with tears flowing now, 'please, I'm sorry, it's too painful – I don't want to talk.' The lady sinks back into her chair, hurt and embarrassed, but I feel victorious. I have said what I have always wanted to say over all the years of my illness: 'It's mine. Don't touch.' Thankfully, the lady is called in to see Dr Jefferson. I sit with my head in my hands and cry. A young man is opposite me. He is so thin and his skin shows the marks of a disease I diagnose immediately. He sits with another slightly younger man who appears very healthy. The older one is dying of AIDS. He leans forward and takes my hand. We sit there, not talking, just weeping and lost in our individual and silent grief. Our eyes meet and we smile. It's okay, his eyes say. It's really not as bad once you get here. I nod at him, understanding, communicating in some strange, unspoken language. There is a camaraderie in our pain. Thanks, I say with my eyes, and give him a mental hug. Thanks, it's just what I needed.

Dr Jefferson tells me to call her Melanie. She explains she is here to help with my symptoms and to offer psychological support. I tell her all about myself – my illness, my family. I tell her how afraid I feel. I tell her about my faith and how I feel this desire to protect my loved ones. She asks me about Richard and how he is coping.

'Denial,' I say. 'He is in denial. He sits up at night working on the computer. It's in our bedroom. Sometimes I wake up and see him, maybe two, three o'clock. Sometimes I just catch him staring and staring at me. But he won't talk to me about it.'

'How does it make you feel?'

'I know how much pain he is in. I really do know how much he loves me. To be honest, I can't think about how he will cope after … after … you know.'

'Who is your best friend?'

'Ellie.' Kindness.

'Is she close to him?'

'Yes, she and her husband, Ian, are close to him. You think maybe he would talk to them?'

'It's worth a try.'

'They could be a sort of link, I guess, between me and him. Another channel of communication.'

'What about the children, Adam and Bethany?'

'It does my head in.' I pause and collect myself. 'Bethany is only eighteen months and I have spent a lot of time away from her with being ill. What is so hard – I keep thinking about it time and time again – she won't even know who her mother was.' I break my heart. 'And

Adam – well, he knows I am ill. And I think somewhere inside he worries about me not getting better. He says his little prayer every night and I just get so scared about how he will be afterwards when I don't get better.'

'Children are very strong, Mary. Usually the children cope better than the adults. And we will be able to help you tell him when you feel the time is right.'

'Yes, but not yet. I want him to have his lovely holiday with me first.'

'Have you thought about anything you could do to help them remember you?'

I shake my head. 'Too scary,' I say, 'but I will begin to think.'

I leave the room shaking. I wish now I had not come alone. I am in pain and tired and so very frightened again. The sweat is pouring off me and my head aches so badly. Ellie works in the hospital so I make my way upstairs to her. I sit in her office and show her my prescription. 'Melanie has put me on these stronger painkillers. They are similar to morphine but with less side-effects. They're called Fentanyl.' I show her the box. 'They are in little patches which stay on for four days. And I can swim with them, too. What do you think?'

'When are you going to start them?'

'Don't know.'

'Mary, it's only a drug.'

'Yeah, but it's a drug that dying people use.'

'Okay, well, let me know because I need to be prepared for when you're off your head.'

'Ellie, we need to plan something else, too.'

'I know. Tell me when you're ready and we'll set a date.'

'And you will look after Richard, won't you?'

'You don't even have to ask.'

Tonight, I am seeing Cathy. She is Compassion. I have something to ask her. Cathy is a psychiatrist and we have worked together for the last three years. I am still worrying about the children and how they will cope with all this. In the aftermath, Richard will become depressed and isolated. I know how he reacts to things. I need her to look after the emotional welfare of my children. I don't want them to end up emotionally scarred or something terrible like that.

Once again, we chat over a meal.

'Do you know, I've never drunk as much champagne as I have in the last few months,' I laugh with my friend. 'Anyway, I have something to ask you. Be serious now.'

208

'It's difficult after a bottle of champagne.'

'It's about my children.' Cath loves children. She hasn't started a family yet but whenever she visits I can see how much she will love them. 'I freak out when I think about them not having a mother. Especially Bethany. Richard is great with them both – truly wonderful. But they still need a mum.'

'Yes, I can understand what you are saying,' Cath says, gently.

'I look ahead and wonder things like who will tell Bethany about girlie stuff and tell her about sex. I want her to have somebody to take her shopping for jewellery and make-up and sit with her when she gets her ears pierced. I want her to know about the womanly side of me – how I looked and how much I loved being totally silly and terribly flirty. I want her to know I wore bright dresses when I was dying and still painted my nails. The sort of stuff only women think about.'

'So how do you want me to help?'

'I have two sisters, Hellie and Franny, plus Ellie and you. I want you to be in charge of Bethany's mother figures. Make sure she has these people in her life and grows up balanced. And please, please tell her about her periods. Help her to buy what she needs. That's your job. And just keep your eye on Adam for me. He is a sensitive little lad.'

Cath looks at me and she is crying. 'I promise.'

'Thank you. I love you.'

'I love you, too.' It doesn't seem peculiar telling my friends I love them. Time is short. They need to know. Love takes away the fear, you see. It takes away some of the pain. We hug and cry and laugh again. Warmth, affection is what I need. I love to feel skin against mine. It means I am still alive. Not a cold, dead body. Not yet.

Only four weeks to go to Australia. Today I am meeting Dafydd.

'Have you ever had lobster?' he asks.

'No, never.'

'Well, that's what we must order. Now, what did you want to ask me about?'

'My conscience is troubling me.'

'Explain.'

'Well, I need to meet my maker with all my past put right. Do you understand?'

'Yes, I do.'

'There are some cases – medical things. I always wondered if I did my best. I feel guilty about them.'

209

'What do you mean?'

'Well, I wonder if maybe I made mistakes that contributed to those patients dying. I need to be free of them. Can I tell you about them?'

'Sure – but remember, Mary, you are only human. We all make mistakes, bad decisions. It's part of the job.'

And so I discuss three cases from my medical career. I recount the details and each time I end up with the questions: 'Was I to blame? Did I under-perform? Was it my fault?' Each time Dafydd reassures me and tells me I was not responsible. I feel my load of guilt ease and I relax, knowing I now have a clear professional conscience.

'I also have a favour to ask you, Dafydd. It's a bit strange.'

'Mary, nothing could be stranger than giving you medical absolution.'

'I want you to speak at my funeral.'

Dafydd looks up from his coffee. 'Why me? I mean, I would be honoured – "delighted" is not the right word – but are you sure I'm the right person?'

'I want you to speak about my life as a doctor. Keep it short – I want a few people to speak about different areas. You are the doctor I always aspired to be. I think, too, that I showed you the best I was capable of. You are the obvious choice.'

'Of course I will, Mary.'

'Keep an eye on Richard for me, Dafydd. I don't want him to go over the edge. He will work himself into an early grave. The kids need him.'

'Don't worry, Mary. We'll keep an eye on him, all of us will.'

We linger over our coffee, knowing time is short, but eventually he has to go and drops me home.

'See you in September then, Mary,' he says, for he is off on holiday tomorrow and then I am going to Australia. We hug each other and I look closely into his serious eyes.

'Perhaps. But if I don't, I need you to know that you played a big part in my life. Truly. You taught me to be a fantastic doctor. I'll never be able to thank you.'

It is the height of summer and July is hot. I am becoming sicker. The pain is getting much, much worse. It is there all the time, boring into my bone, hot and angry. Whichever way I move or lie, it hurts. Eventually my pain overcomes my reluctance to admit I am dying. I carefully apply one of the smallest Fentanyl patches to my skin, hiding it under the edge of my t-shirt. I lie down on the bed in my little boy's bedroom and wait for it to act. I get so tired these days and very weak. I spend a lot of the day resting. It is better in this room, for it is cooler and I am able to watch my tree. It is here, outside the window, beautiful, bright green and with delicate branches. I watch it swaying and bending in the breeze or the birds playing among the leaves where, sometimes, I see a squirrel running along. On a fine day I watch the seagulls circling high on the thermals and on a windy day I watch the clouds racing. I daydream a great deal, thinking about my children, whom I am unable to look after now. Even the smallest task is difficult. I cannot lift Bethany up any more and it breaks my heart. I am too weak to shop or cook or do anything normal. Valerie, my neighbour, who is Calm, brings me meals. Between her and Jan, my childminder, we are managing to cope. Valerie has started coming with me to my hospital appointments, too. She never panics and she makes me feel so at peace. She is a bit like my mum; she smiles with her eyes. She always writes everything down in her little notebook so I can read back over it later on.

I look back on my children's lives and remember special moments. I look forward to their futures and wonder how they will look when they grow up, what sorts of things will make them happy. I remember things in such tiny detail; every sense seems to be sharpened. It is almost as if my mind is making up for my failing body. I listen to my tapes, sometimes classical and sometimes worship songs from church. I lie and soak myself in the music and hope God doesn't mind my rambling prayers because I cannot think very straight. When I doze I curl my hand tightly around the tiny golden cross I still wear around my neck and imagine I am curling up in the enormous hands in the vision of the valley. I picture the waterfall splashing down on my skin and filling me with God's blessings, refreshing me and drenching me in His love. I am not angry with God now. I feel so sad but, in the sadness, I feel very close to Jesus. Sometimes when I awake I know the Presence is there, too, filling the room with light to combat the dark thoughts which would otherwise destroy me.

I talk to God as I rest. I just chat with Him. 'Why?' I still ask. He always tells me to trust Him. To trust Him even unto death. I don't think it is possible for me to be healed now – I am too sick – but I think maybe the healing is in getting through the valley to the enormous hands in one piece. When I pray about my valley now I sometimes see myself on a stretcher: my armour is still on but I am wounded and my

211

fellow travellers are carrying me. I sometimes wonder why I am being carried towards my family. I guess that God must be trying to tell me He will care for them and I will still see them in heaven. I wish though, I do wish, that I could have a little longer. My children are so young, so very young.

So I dream away, peaceful and calm and relaxed. The Fentanyl helps a lot. The pain goes within two hours of putting the patch on and I am able to move more easily. I also feel unaccountably happy. Drug-induced euphoria, I know, but why not? I could do with some help.

Valerie accompanies me to the palliative care clinic where I talk about having goals.

'I need something to aim for each week,' I tell Melanie.

'That's a good idea. Have you thought about doing something for the children yet?'

'I thought about doing a beautiful album. Buying a really special one and telling my life story. I'd like to write some letters to them, too. And I have a book I started to write. I won't finish it, but I want them to know about my life fighting this illness.'

'That's great. Really positive and lovely ideas. How are you feeling otherwise?'

'Well, I feel awful about myself. I look so ill. It makes me feel terrible. When I look in the mirror I see a person with no sparkle.'

'How about artificial sparkle? Make-up, bright jewellery, silly nail polish – that type of thing?'

'Yes, I could try that. I suppose I keep thinking dying people shouldn't look good! Maybe everybody will think I am in denial if I go around all made up.'

'Mary, anybody who is in denial would be unable to confront what you have talked about today.'

'I guess so. I think partly the drugs are making me feel euphoric, but also I feel so terrible that sometimes death seems easier. I have some awful questions to ask today. I am almost too scared to speak them out. I have begun to think about where … you know … where I should go.'

'You mean where you should spend your final time?'

'Yes. I don't want my kids to see me suffering. I don't want them to be scared.'

'A lot of young people choose the hospice for that reason.'

'But what is it like – the hospice? Is it a ward? I would hate to be somewhere really clinical.'

'No, the rooms are like bedrooms with carpets and cosy chairs. We have some family rooms, too, so that Richard could come and stay over.'

'So we would be able to sleep in the same bed?'

'Yes, of course,' laughs Melanie gently.

'I mean, I probably wouldn't feel up to anything naughty, but cuddles are so important, aren't they?'

'Yes, they are. Would you like to visit the hospice?'

Time seems to stop as I contemplate the suggestion. Visit the place where I will die? I don't feel brave enough.

'I couldn't go alone – I couldn't face it.'

'I would be there. You could bring someone – Richard, perhaps?'

'No! No! I don't want him to see the hospice yet. He will have to visit it enough. No, I'll bring a friend. I need somebody detached a little. Somebody clinical. Maybe I could bring a friend and then meet up with my support group afterwards. Have a party to offset the pain. Is that loopy?'

'If it helps you to do it then, no, it isn't loopy.'

'It must be a man, someone strong and someone feel-good …'

I think about the fellow travellers. Courage. I need Courage – he will be perfect for the task. 'Do you think Nigel would mind?' I say.

'I'm sure he won't mind at all.'

That night I ring my friend Sue: Permission.

'Sue, I need you to help me organize something.'

'Another party? I've not got over the last one.'

'No … I need to visit the hospice.' There is a short silence before Sue replies, her voice still bright and cheerful.

'Fine, Mary. Just give me the details and I'll sort it.'

She does. That's what friends are for. Later on she calls back.

'Okay, the Band of Merry Men is sorted. Do it when you come back from Australia. I'll fix a date with whoever you need and we'll be there for you. Then we'll have an almighty party afterwards at my place. Who shall I invite?'

'Just doctors. Can't cope with the explanations. Skill, Endurance, Courage and Permission. Dafydd, Mark, Nigel and you. Okay?'

'Fine, it's sorted. Don't think about it until you come back from your holiday, though.'

'I promise.'

I find a verse from the Bible. The book of Proverbs. 'She is clothed with strength and dignity. She can laugh at the days to come.' I send it to the Merry Men. That is how I want to die.

It is the second week of July. I am so sick. The poison symptoms are terrible. I cannot move without sweating and every movement is a huge effort. Monday morning dawns and Richard has an interview for a consultant's job.

'I can cancel,' he says.

'No. The job is local. It would be what I want most – for you and the kids to be here. I hate to think of you having to uproot Adam and Bethany and taking them away from all that is ours.'

'All right, then. I'll settle you outside with everything you need. If you need help you must ring me straight away on my mobile.'

I lie in the heat of summer under a shady tree. Everything is too big, too sharp. The hedge scents of sweet candyfloss and the wild roses mingle with the brambles. The roses are too big. They are gigantic and so pink and I can see every little wrinkle on the leaves and feel the sharp pain of the thorns even now, before I touch them. Time is distorted. There is too much time but it is running out. I am dying, I know. I am not going to make it to Australia. My goals are contracting, the time is shortening. I am scared, very scared, and I don't want to die. I watch a big bumble bee buzzing around the giant flowers, looking for pollen, and the noise is so loud in my head. Whose life is longer, mine or the bee's? To bee or not to bee. That's funny. Hello, bee. Hello, says the bee and buzzes off. I think I must be dying now. Is this what happens when you die? The noises too loud and the clouds racing by too quickly? I feel the soft grass against my arm and it is so silky and the smell of the earth overwhelms me and I think of the earth and roses on graves. I am going, slipping away into oblivion and there is nobody with me. I don't want to be alone, only me and this bee and the odd passing butterfly. Ouch! Ouch! What is that noise? I'm not on call, am I? It sounds like my emergency bleeper. My mind catches up. The phone is ringing.

'Hi, Mary.'

'Nigel.'

It is Courage. I can hear every noise in the background as if it is right next to me. Nigel is in operating theatre, I can tell. I can hear the water splashing into a metal sink, magnified loudly. I can hear the nailbrush scrubbing against his hands and I can hear the soap bubbles. In the background I can hear a nurse's voice and it is so loud. Turn the volume down, somebody.

'You must be in theatre.'

'Yes, a c-section.'

'Life, new life.'

'Are you okay? You sound strange.'

'Nigel, I think I'm dying soon. Everything is bunching together.'

'Are you feeling unwell?'

'Yes, I feel terrible. Nigel, I'm not going to make it to Oz. I'm so weak and I'm so tired and I feel so ill. I need you to help me, please help me, I'm not ready yet. I don't want to die yet. I want to go to Australia.'

'Okay. Don't panic. Dr Steve Davies, my friend, he can see you tomorrow. He can give you some clever stuff to make you feel better, to stop all these symptoms. Can you make it until tomorrow?'

'I think so. I think I can.'

'Tell me your goals. Come on, what are they? Week by week.'

'This week it's the summer ball.'

'And do you have a new dress?'

'Yes, it's peacock blue and all sparkly. Then, the week after, it's our tenth wedding anniversary. Oh God, oh God, it will be our last one, our very last one.'

'Don't say that, Mary. Shh. Come on. You must not give up.'

'But it's true, Nigel, it's true. I won't see another, will I?'

'No.'

'I'm scared, Nigel.'

'I know you're scared. Come on, what's your next goal?'

'Nothing for that week. I don't think I will make it. I'm dying, I know it, I can feel it. I don't want it to hurt, Nigel, it won't hurt, will it?'

'We won't let it hurt you, okay? I promise. Now, I'm going to ring Steve and then I'll ring you back. Don't die on me, Mary, okay? Don't die on me.'

'I promise.'

Steve is a brilliant doctor. He gives me some tablets to counteract the poison and the effect is absolutely amazing. Within six hours my symptoms begin to improve. What is more, there may – just may – be a way of slowing this tumour down with injections of a hormone called Somatostatin. I'm having a special scan to see if my tumour reacts to it and, if it does, I can have it. All this praying – it is working. Not only do

I feel better but maybe the tumour can be attacked and then I can have more time. The pain has settled a bit, the sweats have gone, I'm stronger and my wheezy chest is better, too. My fingers are still fat but I can live with that! I feel so much better that I am going to the summer ball tonight, which I thought I would have to miss. I have my blue sparkly dress ready and I am looking forward to enjoying myself. I cannot believe how much better I feel and I am sure God is answering my prayers through this new hormone treatment. I knew there would be a breakthrough. I just had to keep trusting. On Tuesday the Elders prayed with me and I was anointed with oil again. We prayed for healing – total clearance from this disease. I think this must be the answer. God is amazing!

Steve also gives me a syringe filled with adrenaline. It is the easy-to-administer type carried on cardiac arrest trolleys. The thing is, the Blob could have a crisis and suddenly decide to chuck a load of histamine into my bloodstream very quickly. If that happens my heart could stop and then the only antidote is the adrenaline. So from now on I need to take my syringe everywhere with me and explain to whoever I am with what to do. It fits rather neatly into my handbag and I show my friends where I keep it. I guess it is a good job that most of them are nurses or doctors and probably could manage to stick the needle in my thigh without fainting at the vital moment. I hope it doesn't happen when I am alone.

The ball is a fantastic occasion. I try really hard to impress. I am sure a lot of the medics are expecting me to look like a skeleton and really ugly. So I spend ages doing my make-up and wear my favourite jewellery. The dress looks gorgeous. 'Tonight,' I tell Richard, 'I want to sparkle. I want to be beautiful. That is how I want to be remembered.'

I arrive at the ball and everybody else is wearing black. It seems ironic that I am sparkly and dying; all the other women are alive but in mourning. I dance all night, whirling and laughing in a haze of Fentanyl and wine. I feel so special, so beautiful. I feel as if I am beyond death. It cannot touch me tonight. Live! Love! Laugh! I think to myself, as the ballroom becomes a fog of smiling and kisses. Hug me and hold me for I am dying and I do not want to believe it. I want to pretend I am Madonna, vibrant, alive and different. I lie on the grass outside the ballroom and look up at the stars. I love everybody! I tell Richard I have this heart full of love and I know I will beat it. This Somato-whatsit will cure me, I know. I'm pinning my hopes on it. It has to work.

'I think you're a bit high, Mary,' warns Richard.

'No, I'm not! I'm just so relieved because I'm going to get well again and I can't believe it! It's amazing, the whole world will be cured of cancer! Awesome!'

A week later is our wedding anniversary. Ten years ago we made our vows. I awaken feeling strangely solemn. It is the last time I shall wake up on my wedding anniversary to breakfast in bed and a huge bunch of flowers. It is the very last time that an anniversary kiss will turn into passionate love-making. Ten years is glass and glass can be fragile …

There is a huge crash and water, flowers and glass end up all over the floor. We look at each other, Hellie and I, our eyes wide with alarm. Time is frozen, for so much is broken …

'Best ever,' I say.

'You always say that, every anniversary,' says Richard.

'That's because it keeps on getting better,' I say.

'Mary Clewlow, I love you for better, for worse … for richer or poorer … in sickness and in health … till death us do part.'

That's when we cry. 'Oh shit,' I cry. 'Oh shit, shit, shit. I don't want to die.'

That evening an open-topped limousine pulls up at the door. It's for me. Blue-sparkly-dress girl. Call me Madonna. I climb in and drink a glass of champagne. And off we go. Over the mountain and the wind is blowing through my hair and I am laughing. I am singing all the love songs there are to sing, including the Beatles favourites I sang to Richard when we became engaged on the Mersey ferry. And I drink my champagne and kiss him in the back of the limousine.

'All you need is love …'

Well, that and your health.

'All you need is love …'

And some time.

'All you need is love …'

I don't want to leave you.

'Love …'

It hurts.

'Love is all you need.'

And a cure, please.

We stand by the lake in Roath Park. The limousine driver pretends not to look at us. My fingers are still like fat sausages and I can no longer wear my original wedding ring. Richard takes out another, bigger gold band he has bought me. In the setting sun, beside the lake, he slips the circle over my ring finger as we renew our marriage vows.

'I, Richard, take you, Mary, to be my beloved wife.'

'I, Mary, take you, Richard, to be my beloved husband.'

'In grave sickness and in failing health …'

'In student debt and in abundant affluence …'

'In the very best …'

'And in the very worst of times …'

'Until we meet again in eternity.'

The bride kisses the groom, who smiles and says: 'How about a honeymoon in Australia?'

'I think I can live with that.'

12

The dive-boat swings gently on the calm turquoise waters of the Coral Sea, still as a millpond under the cloudless blue Queensland sky.

'Are you ready for this?' asks Richard. 'You will always remember your first look on the magical world swimming beneath us.'

Yes, I will always remember. But I will never look upon it again after this trip. This is the last time on the reef for me.

'Let's hold hands and put our heads underwater together, then,' I suggest. So we put on our snorkel masks and, holding hands, we count down 'One ... two ... three!' I plunge my head beneath the surface and my senses are overwhelmed by a myriad of fantastic sights.

Almost as fantastic as the Fentanyl scenes, the drug-induced craziness.

The ocean is crammed with thousands of colourful fish of all shapes and sizes. Through the dense shoals I see the contours of the coral in all shades of pink, orange and purple. I feel the same incredible wonder I felt when I looked upon my newborn son, Adam.

Adam, my son, whom I cannot bear to think of leaving without a mother.

I am overcome with awe at the delicate, magnificent beauty of the world I am floating in. Richard tugs my hand and we dive down to inspect it more closely. The tiny, striped zebra fish seem completely unconcerned by our intrusion. All manner of creatures swim past us. A huge and ugly groper fish lurks near the sea floor. Sea-horses dance and orange jellyfish balloon by. Richard points to a giant sea turtle along the edge of the reef and we spot a manta ray flapping huge wing-like fins. As my head breaks the surface, I am laughing euphorically. 'I've never seen anything so amazing! It's just the most beautiful sight I've ever seen! I can't believe it!'

Nor can I believe I am finally facing death.

'Come on then, mermaid, we have a whole reef to explore!'

This is Heron Island, a coral outcrop and part of the Capricorn Islands on the southern tip of the Great Barrier Reef. It houses huge colonies of seabirds, graceful white herons and millions of very noisy gulls. The trees are literally filled with nests and squabbling birds. The island is a famous honeymoon spot and the luxury resort where we are staying is designed with romance in mind. This has been our second honeymoon, celebrating ten years of marriage. The swimming pools and restaurants overlook deserted white sand beaches. Each evening we have sipped cocktails and watched the sunset's glorious pink perfection.

Tonight, as it darkened, we walked along the beach and lay under the stars, gazing up at the unfamiliar constellations of the Southern Cross and Milky Way. After we made love under the night sky, I sighed contentedly.

'I wish we didn't have to leave tomorrow.'

'I know, but the children will have been missing us. Just think of seeing Adam again and hearing about his Outback adventures.'

'It's so peaceful here. I haven't had to think about ...'

'Shh ... Don't say it, Mary. We're not allowed to talk about it while we're here – we promised each other.'

'I know, it's just I don't want to go back to it all ... I want to stay here on paradise island.'

'Come here, give me a hug and let's watch for shooting stars.' And so we look up at the perfect, velvety sky and count them. Finally, Richard falls asleep and I lie in the warm, scented night and listen to the birds roosting and the giant turtles dragging their clumsy bodies up the beach. I rest my head on my husband's chest and listen to the steady beat of his heart. I wrap my arms around him and hold on to the warmth and certainty of life. I look out into the darkness and feel the familiar fear within me, causing my heart to break with pain.

'Why? Why me? Why now?' I whisper inside my mind, asking the same question I asked so many years ago on the day I first met the Limpet. This time, though, I immediately hear God's answer. I have come to accept it, for what else can I do?

'Trust Me, Mary. Trust Me even unto death.'

Sleepless nights are par for the course now. It is almost as if my body knows time is limited and refuses to miss out. When I do sleep, my mind is filled with strange and bizarre drug-induced sights and sounds. I have learned to calm the fears of the dark small hours and soothe myself by repeating scripture verses learnt by heart. 'Do not be afraid,'

I whisper over and over again until my racing heartbeat steadies and my thoughts quieten once more.

I lie here now looking up at the stars and feeling the gentle, warm sea breeze caressing my skin. Everything seems so intense now that I am living out my final months – it is as if some unknown being has taken what should have been a long life and crammed it into a smaller pot. I have become a concentrated version of myself.

As I lie listening to Richard's gentle, rhythmic breathing I think back to the conversation we had shortly before we left. It was the weirdest week of my life. The week I finalized my plans, just in case I don't make it back from Australia.

It was 28 July 1999, a beautiful sunny day. I was feeling so much better on my special medication and also Blob was not so painful on the new, stronger painkillers.

'What would you like to do today?' asked Richard.

'What I would really love – and I don't know if you will let me – would be to go out for a short bike ride with the children.'

'Do you think you're up to that?'

'No, but I want to go. It might be the last chance for us to go ...'

'Don't say that, Mary.'

'Well it might, we have to face facts. If I take a couple of extra painkillers I will be able to manage if we keep to the flat and don't go too far.'

Richard and I have a tandem bike and we've travelled thousands of miles on it. Our happiest holidays have been on the bike. I have lost count of the times we have wobbled home from a romantic restaurant or slogged up a mountain in a downpour. We always talk best on the bike and that day I needed to discuss one of my worries.

'Richard,' I asked tentatively after the first mile. 'I need you to know something.'

'Go on.'

'It's about after I ... after I die. It's something really difficult to talk about.'

'It's all difficult.'

'It's just ... I want you to know that, after I am gone, I want you to get married again.'

'No! I could never marry anyone else!'

'But you'll be lonely, I know.'

'I'd still be lonely even if I remarried. Nobody could ever live up to you.'

'What about the children? Do you think it would be better for them?'

'Ellie has promised to sort out all the childcare and practical stuff ... and you have your mother-figures. I want it to be just me and the children.'

'But when they leave home you will get lonely and I can't bear to think of you being unhappy.'

'I'll be fine. I'm a bit of a loner, anyway. I'll just immerse myself in work.'

'Sure, and die early too, leaving both our kids without a parent. You need someone to look after you, keep you on the right path. And you need sex. A lot!' We both giggled because our sex life has been just amazing since we discovered I was dying. I guess every cloud has a silver lining.

'I can't believe this – you're not even dead and you're marrying me off!'

'It's because I love you. I want you to be happy.'

'So do you have anyone in mind?'

'Not really. She should be younger, of course, but not more attractive than me. And she would have to love the children totally, as if they were her own. And you must never love her as much as me!'

'How could I? Any other specifications?'

'Yes. She is not allowed to ride this tandem. In fact, she is not allowed to ride any bike with you. I couldn't bear the thought of it. This is my bike and she's not having it. No way! Absolutely no way.'

Richard ground to a halt. 'I can't marry somebody who doesn't enjoy cycling.'

'Richard, she is not having my bike. How could you ever think of it?' My voice became louder as I felt anger rise.

'But Christmas wouldn't be the same without a bike ride.'

'Well, that does it!' I exploded furiously. 'I was kind of thinking that Christmas would be terrible because I was no longer there with you.' I cry easily on this Fentanyl, and I wept embarrassingly loudly.

'Mary, I told you, I don't even want to get married again – you talked me into it. Please don't cry.'

'I'm sorry. I just want you to be happy again one day.'

'Look, Mary, I will never ever get over losing you. Nobody could fill the hole. It's like contemplating ripping my right arm and leg off. It's like we are fused now – one person. How do you replace that? I don't know if it would be fair on this mythical woman who is stealing your tandem.'

Suddenly we both saw the funny side and started laughing hysterically. Adam cycled back with a puzzled expression.

'Why are you laughing so much?'

'Mummy had one of her funny ideas,' replied Richard.

'Oh, is that all? I thought it was something important.' He shook his head at us as we collapsed in laughter again.

It's kind of weird, this dying business. I mean, I imagined I would go round looking completely miserable all the time and everybody would know from my face I was dying. But we still laugh and we still know pleasure and it is almost as if the small joys in life are magnified. If the joy is magnified, though, so is the pain.

Adam's sports day for instance. I lost it – completely. The sun was beating down all afternoon and there we were, cheering Adam in the bean-bag race. The results finally announced, one of the mothers turned to me and said: 'Well, that's it till next year.' That did it. I literally yelled in emotional pain. I was overcome with the grief of losing the pleasure of watching my children grow up. I cried at not seeing Adam in the sack race next year. I wept thinking I would never watch my baby daughter participate in her first sports day. And now it is always the same. Whenever I reach one of my children's milestones, I feel the grief again. The achievements I took for granted I would see now exist only in my imagination. I look at Adam riding his bike proudly without stabilizers and I realize I will not see Bethany do the same. I watch him swim his first length in the swimming pool and know I have taught only one of my children to swim.

Sometimes I wonder how I can be so matter-of-fact. Is my faith sustaining me? Or is the doctor in me taking over and being professional and detached? I guess it is probably a little of both. Take, for instance, 29 July – the day after the tandem argument. Ellie and I arranged to meet. She had a cold bottle of wine, a blanket and a notebook and we headed up to the Wenallt Hill. The evening was a little chilly but the sky was clear and we had a panoramic view over Cardiff. A perfect place for planning a funeral.

'Okay, I want you to know you can tell me anything. I'll write it down and I'll make sure Richard gets to know it all.' We poured the wine, settled on the blanket and began.

'So, first of all – the place?' asked Ellie.

'Rhiwbina Baptist Church, definitely. It's our church family. I need to be somewhere I feel at home.'

'Who do you think should lead the service?'

'David to preach – evangelistic stuff. Along the lines of "if this was you, would you be ready?" Andy Pidcock to lead worship.'

'General theme?'

'Lots of music, lots of flowers and lots of food afterwards!'

'Do you ever stop thinking about your stomach?' laughed Ellie.

'And nobody is to wear black. This is to be a celebration of my life, okay?'

'Yes, but we have to be sensitive, too. Remember your family are going to need some acknowledgement of their grief.'

'So no dancing in the aisles?'

Ellie looked at me sternly. 'Where do we start? Music?'

'Here's a list. All my favourites, starting with a great hymn: "Great is Thy faithfulness ..." '

' "O God, my Father. There is no shadow of turning with Thee." '

' "Thou changest not, Thy compassions they fail not ..." '

' "As Thou hast been Thou forever shalt be!" '

Ellie copied the list into her notebook.

'Which scriptures?'

'Easy – Isaiah. You know the one: "Be not afraid, for I have redeemed you." Then Psalm 91 and then the gospel reading about Lazarus being raised from the dead.'

We arranged everything – the coffin carriers, the order of service and the flowers.

'No horrid purple wreaths, just bunches and bunches of bright flowers.'

'And who is going to speak?'

'Well, I want a few people to speak about different areas of my life. I would like Hellie and Franny to speak for the family. Dafydd is going to speak about me as a doctor, Tim about me as a friend and Brian from Swansea about my Christian life.'

'Sounds good.'

'I would like Nigel to read this poem I have written. And I need somebody to support Richard but I don't know who would be best. Can I leave that to you?'

Ellie wrote some more.

'I'm hungry now. Shall we talk about the rest over a curry?'

'Yeah, why not,' Ellie closed her notebook. We headed to the nearest Indian restaurant and ordered poppadums, onion bhaji and tandoori chicken.

'Do you think this is strange? Arranging a funeral over a curry? Shouldn't I be crying or something?'

'Why? You said it will be a celebration of your life. And, frankly, you will be well out of it by then. I'll be the one with the headache!' We laughed together and then she continued with her scribbling.

'So, what are you going to wear? Your wedding dress?'

'No. I think that would be looking back too much. I want to wear my blue sparkly dress.'

'Please don't be buried in your blue sparkly dress.'

'But I look fab in it. I want to look vibrant!'

'Vibrant? You'll be dead!'

'I insist I wear my blue dress. It's where I'm at now. That's how I want to be remembered.'

'Well, that's very inconvenient.' Ellie looked at me and burst out laughing. 'I wanted to borrow it for the summer ball next year!'

I stared at her for a few seconds and then collapsed in fits of giggles.

'This is hilarious. Surreal – but definitely very funny. You are not – I repeat not – getting your hands on that dress. Oh, and don't forget my make-up and jewellery and whacky nail polish.'

'Which colour?'

'Blue with glitter.'

And that's how we planned my funeral – over an excellent curry. Every detail accounted for. We only cried at one point and that was when I talked to Ellie about the children.

'How do we manage that bit? Are they too young to see me buried?'

'Mary, sorry, but I can't do that bit yet and I don't think you should either. Some things are best left to others.'

Then we both cried and cried and needed to order large brandies. I closed the notebook and gave it to Ellie. She would keep it safe now until it was needed. That's what best friends are for.

I sorted out everything before I left for Australia: the essential letters written, my will updated, the funeral planned and everybody whom I wanted to take part approached. I gave Lydia's box to Ellie to keep safe, for her stuff to be buried with me.

A few days before leaving, I had the worst conversation of all. I told Hellie about the hospice. I hadn't told my family, you see, the outlook.

They knew about the cancer but I hadn't told them it was terminal. I just could not bring myself to do it. All these years I have tried to protect my family from the shadow of the Limpet. I sometimes think it has been harder for my parents than for me to recover from the shocking diagnosis my dad first made. Of course, I never realized at the time, but Dad told me shortly after I qualified that he knew I had bone cancer the second I showed him the lump on my leg, seventeen years ago. How terrible it must have been to diagnose that sickness in his own daughter. He said he felt guilty for diagnosing it, but I said: 'No, you saved my life.'

So Hellie and I sat in the park at the top of the road.

'Hellie, there is something you must know.'

'Don't say what I think you're going to say.'

'I have to. I'm very ill.'

'I know, I can tell. You take so many tablets and all those painkillers.'

'Hellie, you have to be brave. I'm dying.'

We held each other and we cried.

'It's not fair. You've been through so much. You can't die.'

'Hellie – we have to face it, all of us. The family needs to know how ill I am. The bone scan, the Blob – well, that's the baddie. That's the one they can do nothing about.'

'So how long have you got?'

'They can't say. Maybe a few months. I'm getting quite sick now. The tablets are to stop the symptoms but they won't cure me.'

'Isn't there anything they can do – chemo, radiotherapy?'

I explained as simply as I was able.

'So what is happening now?'

I told her about the hospice and seeing the palliative care doctor.

'I can't believe it. You have to be here. We have to be three.'

'Hellie, we shall always be three. In your memory and in eternity, three sisters for ever. But you have to be strong for everybody else.'

'I'm not sure I can be.'

'You have to – for Mum and Dad.'

'Okay, I promise. What can I do? Tell me what can I do!'

'Be there for the children. Love them for me. Love little Bethany as a woman loves a child. I want her to be like you – beautiful and sensitive and female. Look after Adam. He listens to you, respects you. You make him laugh. I need to know they will laugh again. Please, Hellie, you have to do this for me.'

'I promise. And I'll pray every day. I'll pray for you to get better. I don't believe in God, but if He's there I know He will hear me because we know, Franny and I most of all, how much you have fought against it.'

We lay on the grass holding hands and crying. This park is part of our lives. Mum used to bring us here when we were tiny. I remember pushing Hellie on the swings here. It is packed with memories of pain and pleasure.

Jumping through puddles with bright red wellies. Hellie picking daffodils – don't do that, it's naughty. Hide and seek and chase and tag. Franny being brave and Hellie being bossy and me trailing along behind, always shy and cautious. Running races and turning cartwheels and teaching each other somersaults. Playing guitars on the grass and singing and telling each other about boys. A kiss in the dark with Martyn on a cold night and saying no, I'm not ready for that yet. A push in my wheelchair and snowdrops pushing through frozen ground. A dog-walker taking our photograph and staring with pity and my sister swearing under her breath at him. Practising on Lee-Roy and losing my crutches and practising with sticks and then no sticks and then coming up here after Franny's wedding and photographs of sisters three in wedding and bridesmaids' dresses. Pushing the pram with a newborn son and Hellie admiring him, isn't he so gorgeous, you're so lucky, the luckiest woman alive. Then Hellie hugging me as I cried for Lydia, crying for a tiny life sitting under a cherry blossom tree, crying my heart out. Then another pram, a bigger pram, and a tiny, sweet daughter wrapped against the cold. And now we are here talking about hospices and dying.

'Hellie, I love you so much. I love Franny so much. I can't bear to lose you both.'

'I love you, too. Get through, please. I can't live without you. Please.'

'Pray. Let's pray. Come on.'

Tears streamed down our faces as hot and real as in childhood days. Hellie shouted her prayer loudly and desperately.

'God heal Mary. God heal my sister. God, O God, just do it. Amen.'

Amen. We both whispered the word for a long time. Amen.

Four days later we left for Australia. Thanks to Steve's medicine, I felt better than for six months. The symptoms were controlled and the pain better, although not completely gone. I knew the Blob was still there, but at least the poison was being counteracted. I could enjoy this final trip which is so important to me.

We walked off the plane into a Queensland winter – perfect blue skies and 28°C. Adam's eyes widened as he saw palm trees swaying and brightly coloured parrots.

We headed straight for Bundaberg, Adam's birthplace and the home of our medical school friend, John Wakefield. As we drove through fields of sugar cane and paw-paw groves, Adam's voice became more and more excited. We turned a corner and saw the hospital, just as we had left it.

'That's where you were born!'

It was like walking back in time.

'This is where Mum and Dad worked and here is the ward where you were born.'

The midwives remembered us and admired the lively six-year-old they saw enter the world in 1992. Nothing had changed and yet so much had changed for us. The reason for our trip was known only to our close friends here. My heart was cut through as I looked at Adam in his carefree enjoyment and remembered this was our final trip. John had given us the use of his beach-home while we were here. It was the same house in which we had stayed before. The memories came flooding back as we sat by the azure swimming pool in the balmy night.

'We sat here the first night we came to Australia,' I told Adam. 'You were a tiny jelly baby, only a few centimetres long, in Mum's womb.'

'And I made you feel very sick, didn't I?'

My heart broke again as I looked at his perfect trusting innocence, and I shuddered as I considered what lay ahead for him.

'Yes, you did – you and Bethany! I sat by this pool and I just could not believe I was having a baby.'

'And then where did you go next?'

'Wait and see …'

'This is it, Adam. This is the Outback,' I told him, as we stopped beside a dirt road, miles from anywhere. His eyes took in a seven-foot cactus and a huge termite mound. He spotted some kangaroos and a flock of cockatoos and ran quickly into the bush after them.

'Stop there, Adam! There could be snakes!'

His eyes widened in alarm as he realized the hazards of Outback life. 'You must be careful here,' I said. 'Big snakes hide in the bush.'

'Could they kill me?'

'Yes, they could.'

'Scary!'

Yes, very scary, my child. Death is very scary and I am afraid for you, frightened to lose you, terrified of leaving you.

It was as if we had never left. We strolled into the tiny hospital at Eidsvold with Adam in tow. Vera was bent over some paperwork and looked up. We had not warned her of our visit.

'I guess this is Adam, then?' she said, calmly, as if this happened every day. We talked and talked, catching up on six years.

'I've been thinking about you a lot over the last few months,' Vera said, suddenly. 'You've been on my mind a lot. You okay?'

'Not really, Vera,' and I told her the story.

'You'll be right,' she said. 'I've always known it. You'll make it. Sometimes you just have this feeling.'

I hugged my friend and we set off deeper into the Outback to the home of our Australian friends, Chris and Janelle Homan. Seven years have passed and five children have been born since we last met. It was as if the intervening years had never separated us.

'You two need some time together,' they told us. 'Quality time, romance, no kids. How would Adam enjoy being an Outback kid for a few days? You two head off to the reef.'

So that is how we came to be here, romancing on Heron Island. We took up their offer and booked a second honeymoon in a tropical paradise. Time to recover a little, time to laugh. Time to snorkel the beautiful Barrier Reef together and swim in the calm Coral Sea. But, most of all, time to enjoy a love for which time is now running out.

How can I describe how I feel tonight, lying here in a tropical wonderland wrapped in the arms of my lover? Still bodies entwined in the darkness, lives so enmeshed that I do not know where I finish and Richard begins. My eyes will not cry as I think of all that this life, this love, means to me. Our special moments and times, the memories of all we have shared. I catch his scent on the breeze.

A box with a skeleton and can I help you? A bench on a ferry and a sixties song. A lilac ballgown and holding him tight. Walking hospital wards, lectures and long nights poring over books. The first time we kissed and the first time we argued and the first time we made up and the first time we made love. The joy on his face as he got down on his knees and gave me an emerald ring. I love you, Dr Clewlow, and I love you, Dr Self. May I carry your skeleton again? Layers of cream silk and a veil lifted back. A bed of pink roses which he lifted me on to and gently took off my wedding dress. The long, long nights of being a doctor and coming home to strength and a cuddle. Seeing the pink dot and knowing we were having a baby and Adam all newborn-slimy and Richard kissing him. My son. A proud smile. Then tears. I'm losing her, Richard. Our Lydia. Shh, don't cry. I'm here, I'm always here. And he is. Bethany next – tiny in big strong arms and exhaustion and pain and loving me in all that blood and gore and everything that is childbirth. Then the Penny, the terrible Penny, and waking from madness and finding him there and feeling safe. And seeing the Blob and crying together and knowing the worst and soothing hugs and tender caresses and all that is us. So much that is us and I do not know how I can leave him. I do not know how I can bear him being cleaved away from my heart and I am crying and shaking with the unfairness of it all. Until he wakes, holds me tight, wipes my tears, kisses my face on our last night on Heron Island and we are lost in the pain and despairing, frantic passion once more.

The next morning we collect Adam. He has had a great time playing with his new friends and becoming an Aussie boy in our absence. He walks round proudly, barefoot, in his baseball cap and shades, pointing out the Outback wildlife. It is a tearful parting from our friends. It is unspoken, but we are unlikely to meet as a foursome again.

'Mary, be strong,' urges Janelle. During our visit we have become godparents to their six-month baby, Claudia. I hide my face in the milky bundle.

'I will, I promise. Goodbye. It's meant so much to us being here and seeing you again. Thank you for asking us to the christening – that has been so special.'

'It is special to us, too.'

'Make sure you tell her all about me, won't you.'

Janelle holds me tight and we both cry. We all wave until their home is well behind us.

Several hours later we reach the ferry and collect the four-wheel-drive vehicle that we need to use on the next stop on our Australian tour: Fraser Island, the biggest sand island in the world. Adam is overcome with excitement to ride in the army Land-Rover and he sits between us, waving to ferry operators. The roads on Fraser Island are sand tracks and the vegetation thick, verdant rainforest. Parrots and birds of paradise hide in the canopy and crystal-clear lakes lie hidden deep in the forest. We visited here once before, when I was heavily pregnant with Adam, and we laugh now as we tell him the story. It is the most breathtakingly beautiful place I have ever seen.

'So, the last time we came here, you were still in Mum's womb.'

'How fat were you?'

'Very fat. It was about two months before you were born.'

'I bet I didn't like all the bumps,' Adam giggles.

'No, you did not, and every time Dad went over a very big bump you kicked Mum under the ribs! In fact the roads were so bumpy we thought you were going to be born here!' Richard and I laugh as we reminisce about the last night we spent on Fraser Island, almost seven years ago.

'I'll never forget you waking me up at two o'clock in the morning.'

'Yes and I'll never forget the hour before that, lying wide awake and wondering how on earth you were going to deliver a premature baby in a tent on a deserted island!'

'I'm having contractions – that was the last thing I wanted to hear!'

'Well, it wasn't much fun for me either, you know! Anyway, thank goodness the contractions settled down.'

'So was I almost born here? On this island?' Adam is giggling at the story too.

'We did think you might be, but then you stopped wanting to be born and we headed home the next day!'

'We used to do some crazy things, didn't we?' says Richard.

'Yes, we did. I guess I always had that feeling of wanting to live life as fully as possible – in case. Whizzing down the Ardèche Gorge on the bike at sixty miles an hour, climbing glaciers in New Zealand, swimming in Loch Ness on New Year's Eve! I have no regrets. How I wish I had a bit more time to do crazy stuff.'

We picnic by the edge of Lake Mackenzie. The water is cold and clear. We teach Adam to snorkel in the shallows. I tread water and watch his first attempt and feel so grateful I have known the love of my firstborn. In the bright sun, against the backdrop of the rainforest, I remember his milestones. I see him as a baby nestling in my arms, his head close against my breasts and his tiny fists curled up tight. I see him as a toddler, picking up coloured stones on the beaches of the Gower. I remember him taking unsure steps on his first birthday, face covered in chocolate and hands outstretched to me. So much to remember … his first words, the first snowman he made and hanging out his first Christmas stocking. Bringing home messy three-year-old's paintings, and then his first day at school, proudly dressed in his smart new uniform. I taught him to read his first word and to turn his first somersault. I remember him sitting in Nigel's room, watching the baby appear on the scan. It's my sister! he said. Then came the day when he crept into my hospital room with big wide eyes and peeped through the side of the cradle. She is so cute and so tiny, he said, and never a moment of jealousy, just protectively watching out for her and kind cuddles when she fell. His first sports day and his first nativity, his first report and the first of everything else that I have not seen and never shall. My heart is grieving and I long so much to be there for his first girlfriend and his first exams. I long to see what he will become. I long to see him for a little longer. But it shall not be.

'Mum, why are you crying?'

'It's just the sun making my eyes water.'

'Come on and watch my first dive.'

The days fly by in a whirl of exploration. All too soon, our adventure is over and we return to the sunshine coast of Queensland to relax on the beaches. The trips have tired me and my symptoms have worsened again. I double up the dose on Steve's treatment and rest in the sunshine. The last few days are spent splashing around in the pool with Adam. More tearful goodbyes as we leave and head back to Brisbane to catch our flight home. There are so many goodbyes.

'Goodbye, Australia!' calls Adam as we take off. I close my eyes and fight back the tears. I do not want to return to tests and treatment and uncertainty. Goodbye, Australia. Goodbye to a part of my life that was lived free of the Limpet, the Penny and the Blob. Goodbye to my dear friends and goodbye to the Barrier Reef. My final trip is complete and what a trip it was. And this will be my last homeward flight.

We return to Cardiff. It is early September. It is not long before I am back in hospital clinics and back down to earth. First, I go to see Steve in the endocrinology unit. The special scan to see whether I can have Somatostatin should have been analysed. I am so hopeful of this treatment, but the news is not good.

'The secondary doesn't react to the Somatostatin. There is no benefit to having the hormone treatment.'

I sit outside the hospital with my head in my hands. Valerie is with me. I am crying again. I am always crying. The news is always bad.

'What am I going to do? Every time I come here the news just gets worse. I was pinning my hopes on this stuff and now it's all for nothing. My hopes get dashed time and time again.'

There is nothing to say. Valerie waits until the storm subsides.

'I'm losing hope, Valerie. I really do think now I am going to die. It's terminal.'

A few days later my fears are reinforced when I visit Professor Mason, the oncology expert. There is no treatment. Bone secondaries kill you. That's all there is to it. He is so kind and helpful in every way, but even he cannot halt the advance of the rebellious army which is killing me. I have access to the best doctors but I am still dying. The darkness of despair descends and my hope begins to die.

I am in the palliative care clinic again. There is a black question I must ask. I cannot speak it to anyone except Melanie. After we have confirmed the hospice visit, I broach it.

'Melanie, I have an awful question to ask.'

'Fire away, then.'

'When I die … What happens? I mean, before the actual dying bit. Does it hurt? Will I know what is happening?'

Melanie explains. As the pain gets worse, I will need more and more Fentanyl and morphine and eventually I will just be asleep all the time. I won't be in pain. I won't be conscious. I won't remember. When Richard holds my hand and sits by my bed I won't know. When my kids come and kiss me I will not recognize them. When last goodbyes are said I will not be there.

How do I get my head round that?

I soon discover how much pain the Blob can cause. It is a Saturday morning, two weeks after our return from Australia. My tree has turned golden yellow as the autumn begins. I am feeling tired and weary. My symptoms are terrible and the pain is getting worse. Richard has taken the children out for the day and left me to rest. Usually I doze peacefully but today the pain does not ease. I take the maximum amount of painkillers. It still hurts a lot. I try some sedatives but I still cannot settle. I try everything I can think of – distraction, a bath, a hot-water bottle. The pain gets worse every hour. Soon I am in agony and I am scared. Is this it? I think it is. I am alone again. I am not ready. I have not said my farewells. I call Ellie and end up in the doctor's surgery. By now I am rolling round in agony. The pain involves the nerves now, I know. I feel as if I am giving birth. 'I need to push,' I keep telling Dr Edwards, my general practitioner.

'It's the nerves in your pelvis. They must be inflamed. I think you need to go in for pain control.'

'No! No! I'm not going to the hospice. I'm not going. I'm still too scared. I haven't visited it yet. I didn't think it would be so soon.'

'But you need to go in, really, Mary. This pain is unbearable for you.'

I scream again as another bout takes hold. I am writhing and rolling. I do not care. It hurts, I keep saying, it hurts.

'Who can I contact? What about Richard? We need someone to decide where you can go.'

'Richard has taken the children out for the day. I'm not going to the hospice.'

'Okay, you're panicking. Who else knows about your care?'

'Ring Nigel.'

A few minutes later, Dr Edwards puts down the phone. 'It's sorted. Melanie will take care of you on Nigel's ward in gynaecology.'

'Okay, okay, just get rid of this pain.'

I lie on the crisp white hospital sheets and Ellie soothes me. 'Richard is coming now. You'll be okay.'

I am crying and writhing, waiting for the pain control doctor to visit me. I cry with relief when Richard walks through the door followed by a colleague. Richard gives me a hug and then takes hold of my arm. He turns. 'I'll put her drip in,' he says, 'she gets scared.'

I do not feel a thing as Richard hits my vein first time. I say to him through gritted teeth: 'Better than Dr Tan-Shoes.'

'And this is better than a double brandy,' says Richard as his colleague draws up a large dose of morphine. I am kicked into silence with a euphoric rush of absence of pain.

'Oh God. That's wonderful. Better than sex.'

Push the button when you need, it gives you the drug, and so I do when it hurts, and then I start to laugh. The night passes and the drug just keeps on making me laugh. Lots and lots of lovely morphine floating on a nice fluffy cloud and smiling at everybody because I do so love them. Hello everybody, I love you all. This is so lovely, this dying and sleeping bit cocoons of safety. The pillows are soft and this is my womb and I can die here it's nice.

Hi, Melanie, it was hurting me a lot but now it's not so bad and hello Nigel I love this ward and actually I love everybody I really do. Look at my pictures of Australia. I'm going back there when this is all over when I'm cured and when the whole world is cured of cancer. Where do I put this patch, it's bigger isn't it more Fentanyl yes please and more morphine too it's just like a party do you want to come to my party the patch is lovely and makes me feel great.

Hello, Ellie, I'm dying but that's cool, you know what I want. I want the Elders. I could still get healed, you know, look after the children I miss them you brought my photos put them where I can see them I love them I miss them oh no I'm crying now. If I'm not healed completely I want to die, I can't go on, send me some people, links with my life, not heavy just links. Ruth because of Lydia and Margaret because of work and Mark to look after Richard.

My Merry Men phone. Be brave says Dafydd be brave says Sue, Nigel visits me every day sometimes he looks so sad why does he look so sad. Richard dear Richard is always here back and forth bringing me goodies and lovely flowers. But I miss the children I can't let them see me dying but I miss them and I kiss the photograph and cuddle Ad's teddy and Beth's dolly. I can smell them, you see, on their toys I can smell every part of my sweet boy's skin and my musky girl's hair.

Night falls. Strange things are happening again. Not scary just strange. A little procession of dwarves enters my room and I sit up hello dwarves hello Snow White. But I'm not I've done bad things maybe I'll go to hell. They march around the room singing hi ho hi ho. There are three little dwarves at the back and they are looking at me a boy dwarf and two girls I know them. Adam! Hello Adam he looks at me and waves and the procession is walking out of the door no! no! don't leave me. Adam is waving goodbye and he is leaving and then I see the littlest dwarf she skips out after Adam and turns as she leaves the room and waves shyly and I see it is Bethany. And now there is only one little dwarf, a middle-sized one, she is wearing white and has a set of glittery wings. She flies up onto my bed and sits there who is this? I look at her face and she smiles and says Mummy. She looks like Hellie all dark hair and white teeth. Lydia! It's Lydia! Hello my darling girl I never ever thought I would set eyes on you so this must be heaven and I must be dead. Lydia places her soft little hand in mine and it is all plump and perfect but her lips are blue and she must have had a bad heart but now she is mended and here. Don't be frightened Mummy go to sleep have a sweetie don't cry and she gives me one of her jelly babies to make me better.

Hello Ellie there were dwarves in my room last night and they were so cute. Lydia was there too. What would I like? I'd like some jelly babies lots of them a massive big box of them that's all I want. Let's sing some songs because I'm so happy I really am I might be dying but I am very happy. Come on don't be embarrassed. I just want to praise the Lord for all that He has done for me, one, two, three, shine Jesus shine fill this land with the Father's glory. It's not too loud don't be silly we are meant to be witnessing to the nurses.

Hello Margaret thanks for the jelly babies would you like one? I'm coming back to work soon did you know you must tell them all I'll be back soon. I'm going to be cured and the whole world will know and it will be awesome. The jelly babies must contain some special anti-cancer drug I've discovered the secret cure soon the whole world will hear of my amazing recovery and it will all be because of jelly babies.

Hello Elders what are you doing here? You've come to pray with me is that medicine? Oil? This nurse will sit with me and then you can pray wise men praying and dabbing oil on my head and it's lovely and peaceful and I feel all warm and where is the Presence is he here too I cannot see him but I can feel him around here somewhere. I have this scan tomorrow to see the tumour and I don't think I'm going to get well and I'm going to another hospital in Birmingham maybe they know something that these doctors don't know maybe they can cure me do you think they can cure me do you think God can cure me I do hope so because if not I'm stuffed.

'Hi, Ellie, I feel a bit better today.'

'Great. I think it's because the morphine has been stopped and now you are just on Fentanyl patches – the strongest dose.'

'Have I been hallucinating again?'

'Just a bit. But it should settle down now. Have you any pain?'

'A little, but nothing to speak of, really.'

'Well, now the pain is controlled we need to get you transferred to Birmingham – to the Royal Orthopaedic Hospital.'

'To the Bone Tumour Unit?'

'Yes, Professor Mason and Nigel have been sorting out the referral for you. I think you are going there on Monday. It's Thursday today. If your pain is controlled you should be able to go home for the weekend.'

'Do you think that maybe they will be able to do something – surgery or anything to give me longer?'

'One step at a time. You've been crazy for the last three days.'

'Did I do anything embarrassing this time?'

'No, but you did eat the most enormous box of jelly babies in record time!'

'Compared to talking fish tanks, I guess that's pretty mild!'

Ellie helps me wash and comb my hair. She hands me a mirror. I look at my reflection. My skin is covered in tiny marks. It looks as if my skin is dying. My hands are the same. The skin is damaged. My face is swollen and puffy and I feel so ugly. I am so weak and so very tired.

'Ellie, I'm ready to go. I can't go on.'

'Shh. Let's see what they say in Birmingham.'

I am discharged on Friday to spend the weekend at home and then I will be admitted to the Bone Tumour Unit in Birmingham. Nigel calls in before I leave. I am sitting on the bed and Richard is holding my hand.

'I've come to say cheerio and I hope Birmingham goes well. Tell me how you get on.' He stands for a long time at the end of the bed, watching Richard and me. He has a peculiar look on his face. I feel scared. I have seen the look before.

As he walked away down the ward I suddenly realized why he had come and why he looked at me so strangely. He thinks I'm going to die ...

'I'll be okay, Nigel. I will.' He nods and leaves as Ellie enters.

'Nigel thinks I'm going to die in Birmingham,' I tell her.

It is 21 September – a week since I left the University Hospital in Cardiff. I have been waiting for the doctors to call me to the Bone Tumour Unit. I expected it to be a big shiny modern building, but the Royal Orthopaedic Hospital in Birmingham is a warren of corridors and a misshapen collection of ageing buildings. Richard and I make our way to Ward Twelve.

I have been asked to arrive prepared to go to theatre, so I have not eaten since last night. The oncologists want to biopsy the Blob. I change into my pyjamas and rest on the bed. Richard leaves to return home and care for the children. Within ten minutes the porter is knocking on my door and a nurse arrives.

'Time to go down for your operation,' she says. I feel bewildered and scared. I have only just arrived. I don't know anybody. What if I should die under the anaesthetic surrounded by strangers? I am alone. A nurse applies some tape to my wedding ring to cover it up and quickly puts an identity bracelet around my wrist.

'I am not alone, though,' I think to myself. 'God is at my right hand. He will be with me.' I recite the words of Psalm 23 to myself as I did when I had my thoracotomy. The anaesthetist greets me cheerfully in the operating theatre. It feels strange to be in a hospital where I do not recognize all the names and faces. As the anaesthetist draws up the drug to send me off to sleep, I am struck by a terrible thought. I do not want to wake up again. And yet I do not want to die alone. Soon I let go of consciousness and sink into black oblivion and I think I am crying as I fall asleep.

I awake to a noise of clatter and crashing. An orderly pops her head around the door of my side ward.

'Hello, you're awake now. Would you like a sandwich?'

I take off my oxygen mask and try to work out where on earth I am. 'Where am I?' I could be in any of the many hospitals I have seen in my short life.

'Ward Twelve.'

'No, I mean which hospital?'

The orderly laughs. 'They gave you a good anaesthetic. It's the Royal Orthopaedic.'

Now I remember! My bag is still unpacked by the bedside. I try to sit up. 'Ouch! My back hurts!' The orderly leaves a plate of sandwiches on my table and rushes off to find the nurse.

'Hello, Mary. I'm the sister on the Bone Tumour Unit. Sorry it was such a rush into theatre!'

'That's okay. At least it's over now. What time is it?'

'Tea-time. You've been snoozing away all afternoon. Mr Grimer and Dr Spooner from our team will be here to see you shortly.'

'The orthopaedic surgeon and the oncologist, right?'

I recognize the names from letters I have received. I know they are experts in the field of bone tumours occurring in childhood; Mr Grimer, in particular, has a growing worldwide reputation. The nurse explains a little about the unit as she checks my wound.

'That looks fine,' she says. 'Try and eat your sandwiches and have a drink, then you should be able to go home to Cardiff once the doctors have been.'

Several hours later, two doctors enter the room. They shake hands with me and I tell them my story. They spend some time looking at my charts and my notes before they explain their ideas.

'Well, Mary,' begins Mr Grimer, who is very tall and younger than I expected, 'you have been causing us a lot of headaches.'

I laugh. 'That's par for the course with me, I'm afraid. My nickname in Cardiff is Heartsink!'

'We have been taking a look at all your notes and tests. We have also checked your operation biopsies from both the lung tumour and your original bone tumour. We sent for the slides from Blackpool.'

'And what do you think?'

'This will come as a surprise to you. You had – indeed have – an incredibly rare type of bone cancer. So rare that anything I say is guesswork.'

'But I thought I had an osteosarcoma?'

'No. What you had is a type of tumour called a mesenchymal chondrosarcoma.'

'Never heard of it.'

'You wouldn't. It has only recently been identified as a separate disease.'

'What does it mean for me?'

'Well, it explains why you have relapsed so late – this tumour can relapse after twenty years. It also explains why it has been behaving so strangely: it is a most bizarre type.'

'How rare is it?'

'Well, we have seen one thousand osteosarcomas here. But we have only ever seen five tumours like this. Hence my point that it is an unknown entity.'

'So does that mean it is curable?'

'No … but we might get you some remission time if we use a combination of chemotherapy and radiotherapy.'

'Can't you remove it surgically?'

'If we did, it would involve the most radical surgery – we would have to remove half your pelvis and that would leave you wheelchair-bound. It could also damage your pelvic nerves.'

'Leaving me incontinent?'

'Almost certainly.'

'No – no, I am not having that, no way. My life would not be worth living.'

Mr Grimer nods sympathetically. 'I know. I have to explain, though.'

'You do understand I've got two kids? If I cannot be independent then I don't want to be alive.'

'Which leaves us with chemotherapy and radiotherapy.'

'The chemotherapy would be VIPA, yes?' I recall with horror the side-effects.

'I'm afraid so.'

239

'The radiotherapy would be pretty localized to my pelvis so we would be talking radiation damage to my ovaries and I'd be menopausal?'

'Yes, I'm afraid so. There would also be damage to your bladder and bowel because the tumour is so close to those organs.'

'But that wouldn't make me incontinent?'

'No. The point is, we really don't know how much benefit this would give you. We are working on very limited experience. There are no right and wrong answers. It is a choice you need to make.'

'But we are talking about buying time? The tumour won't disappear?'

'We are talking time.'

'I need to think about it for a while. Is that okay?'

'Of course. We will see you in clinic in a few weeks and perform another CT scan.'

I return home depressed and despondent. Everything has changed once more. I have to think about active treatment again. There are no proper answers and the uncertainty is awful. What is more, I have now seen world experts and one thing is certain: I am never going to recover from this illness. It has been confirmed three times now. The best doctors in the world cannot cure me. There is no surgery, no drug, nothing powerful enough to halt Blob the bastard. I hate it, I hate it.

Blackness descends. I try to hide my feelings from those close to me. I go to one of the Elders, Alan, and tell him how things are looking.

'Basically, I am dying but I don't know when and I don't know whether or not I should have this treatment. It could kill me anyway and nobody can tell me if it will buy me much more time. I am so confused. I am so depressed. I need some answers.'

Alan and his wife, Ceri, listen carefully. 'Okay,' Alan says, 'we need to mobilize everybody in prayer. We need to get everybody praying and fasting. This is desperate now. We need a breakthrough.'

'I feel so ill, too. I either want to die soon or get better completely.'

'Come to the Elders' meeting and be prayed with again and we'll anoint you with oil. We'll also set aside a day for prayer and fasting to ask for your healing. Maybe we could contact other churches, too.'

The following day I am anointed. The Elders pray and Ceri puts the oil directly onto my bone tumour. Nothing happens and the next day I feel exactly the same. A week later many churches spend the entire day in prayer and fasting for my healing. In an idle moment I list the churches where I know people are praying for me. It occurs to me that ten thousand people worldwide are praying for my recovery. I wait at home all day, expecting to feel better but, if anything, I feel worse. My asthma worsens and any slight exertion causes my body to become soaked with sweat. I am still in pain, even with the strongest Fentanyl patch, and I am so weak. I try to pray but I feel hopeless inside. I read my Bible but the words seem empty. I cannot understand why God does not hear me.

'What are you playing at, God?' I ask Him angrily.

'Trust Me even unto death,' He replies.

Fine. I'm dying. God hasn't healed me. After all these years of being faithful and following the Lord, He does not care about me. So what? I'm sick of it all. The praying didn't work. The anointing didn't work. The fasting didn't work. All the Bone Tumour Unit has come up with is a living death regime. What have I done, hey, to get all this garbage thrown at me? So I'm angry. Well, I think I'm entitled to be angry. I am absolutely furious. Mostly at God. As far as I'm concerned, God can get lost. It is now eight months since my relapse. Eight months of praying every day. Eight months of trusting. Eight months of pain, fear and confusion. And how is this rewarded? Surprise – I'm still dying. Every time I ask God to heal me He just ignores me. He did it when I was seventeen and He's doing it now. So now I shall do it in my own strength. Not that I have much strength left. I shall just enjoy myself and forget about death and forget any hopes of healing. It's all stupid lies, anyway. God doesn't love me. If He did He wouldn't allow this to happen. All He says to me is trust Me unto death. What good is that? I don't want to die – that's the whole point. So I'm not going to trust Him. I'm giving up on Him. I don't need Him. I've got friends, the best doctors in the world. I'll do it myself. I don't need any help from God who, frankly, I no longer believe exists.

It is 4 October. Tonight I am going out with the Merry Men. We are all going to Cardiff Bay. Strength, Courage, Feel-good: that's what I need. None of this God stuff. I am going to get absolutely legless – excuse the pun – as I have been doing every night for the last week. At least if I'm drunk then I don't hurt. I know what you're thinking. It's wrong and I shouldn't do it. Well, who cares? I'm dying, aren't I? I'm not hurting anybody. And it's not as if I'm going to die of cirrhosis first. So don't even think of judging me unless you have been where I am. Dying. Angry. Let-down. There is a blackness in my mind and my heart. I have lost my hope and I have lost my soul. My day is spent in bed. My night is spent in bed – after I've drunk a couple of bottles of wine, that is. The sole delight in my day is the two hours when Richard comes home and helps me cuddle the children. I can't do anything for them, of course – can't even change Bethany's nappy. I mean, it is really sad when the one thing you want to do is change a nappy. How I wish I could do that for my baby. But I can't. The children sit on my lap and I cuddle them. I sing to Bethany and listen to Adam read. That's it. That's my day. Then Richard goes into denial and I go into denial. He studies, I drink. The four-day Fentanyl patch still makes me feel high and happy but only on the first day. The rest of the time I just feel ... out of it. I haven't told anybody about the drinking or losing my faith. What's the point? What can anyone possibly say to help me? I'm thirty-four, I have two children and I'm dying. Why? There is no answer.

So I dress up in all my best gear. Pretty black dress with sparkly bits, make-up, jewellery, lacy underwear. Stick on a new Fentanyl patch and off I go. Cardiff Bay here comes Madonna. I am meeting the Merry Men in one of the smartest restaurants in town. By the time I get there the Fentanyl has kicked in and I am euphoric.

'Hello, everybody!'

'You look great!'

'Well, dying is no excuse to look miserable, now is it?'

I can't believe I just said that. I feel totally desperate, deep down inside. Scratch the surface and it is black underneath. If only they knew.

'Wine? Yes, please!' I drink and somebody fills it up and I just keep drinking. Sometimes I swop glasses round and soon I lose count of how much. Still, nobody can tell because I am always very silly on the Fentanyl and all my friends will just assume it's the drugs.

My mind begins to do very strange things. I truly am dying and I need to be rescued. But there is nobody powerful enough to do it, is there? No, nobody. Perhaps I can escape on my own because I am trapped in a body and scared so scared of dying. I feel terrible and nothing takes it away. My mind is empty my thoughts are disappearing. My body is dying and soon I will be gone from here and my two babies and my lover will remain and I will be nowhere because now I do not even know if there is a God any more and if there is He doesn't love me or why would He do this? I cannot breathe I feel so scared and I just want to go go away go anywhere escape and be alone. Where will I go if there is no heaven and no God? The worms will eat up my body and I will become part of a cherry blossom tree and then I will be chopped down one day and bulldozed away. It is horrific, this dying thing. It is unknown and I cannot do it. I am fighting to stay, fighting to remain, but I don't have the strength to fight any more. I just want to be rescued please rescue me. I need some air and I am walking out of the restaurant and into the night. The wind cuts me through and I am cold in my thin dress but it doesn't matter nothing matters any more and I am nothing. Sit down by a flower pot and shiver. Shiver with fear and shiver with cold and shiver with fear of being cold and dead and dead and cold. I lie down because I am tired and I may as well get used to the ground because that is where I shall soon be. If I lie here maybe I shall die and it will be taken away from me. I hear a noise the sound of chinks. What is it? It sounds like skeletons dancing. I am so scared they are coming for me death is coming for me and it is not right that I am here alone and lying on the ground. I look at the moon and it is big and pale and white the water laps against the water-break I cannot leave them I cannot. My children. Tiny Bethany and funny Adam. I think of their warmth. But I still feel cold. What is the noise? Dancing skeletons. No-one is going to rescue me close your eyes Mary close your eyes and when you wake up you will be in the ground. Dead.

'Ellie?'

'Mary?'

'Oh, Ellie,' I sob into the phone.

'Where are you and what time is it?'

'It's three o'clock in the morning and I'm sitting on the garden wall.'

'Where have you been?'

'I fell asleep on the Bay. The police found me and were concerned for my safety and brought me home.'

'Why were you asleep on the Bay?'

'I drank too much. It interacted with the Fentanyl. I just felt totally desperate and lost it, I suppose. I sat down by this flower pot and thought I could hear skeletons but it was flagpoles and then I woke up and it was two o'clock and everybody had left the restaurant.'

'So do your friends know where you are?'

'No, I don't think so.'

'Is Richard home?'

'Yes, but I don't want to tell him I've been drinking so much.'

'Tell him. You must. You must tell him how you feel.'

'Ellie, I'm so scared. I don't want to die.'

'I know. Go inside, wake Richard and we will talk tomorrow. Don't worry, we'll sort it.'

'Do you still love me? You're not mad at me, are you?'

'Mary, I love you and I'm not mad. Now go to bed!'

I wake Richard and tell him about the drinking and the madness and being angry at God. I tell him I love him and love the children and cannot bear to think of dying. He holds me while I cry for a long time and then tucks me up and soothes me to sleep.

The following morning I meet with Ellie. I have a terrible hangover.

'I'm sorry,' I cry. 'I said sorry to Richard, too.'

'Hey, it's okay,' she says calmly. 'So you lost it. You're dying. Everybody loses it sometime. Let's put it right now and sort you out.'

'It's because I felt angry with God, so I turned my back on Him. I told Him to get lost.'

'I'm sure God is big enough to take it.'

'My faith – it's all I have to hold on to, isn't it?'

'Well, it does look like it. The doctors can't cure you.'

'But I feel so let down that God isn't healing me. I guess I am fighting Him. I want my own way, and if I don't get it … then I get mad.'

'What about this drinking. How much have you been drinking?'

'A lot. Maybe two bottles of wine a night – only for the last week, though.'

'Well, that was a great idea when you're taking all that medication too.'

'Oh come on – I'm dying. Give me a break, please.'

'It doesn't make it okay, Mary. And let's face it – has it solved anything?'

'No, but I'm sure God must understand.'

'Well, He does, but He still wants you to rely on Him, not anything else. Not alcohol and not other people. It's you and Him.'

'So what do I do?'

'I think you need to get back to where you were when you said if you were healed it was great, but if you weren't then it was still okay.'

'You mean I need to trust Him even if He doesn't heal me? Even if I don't get my own way?'

'Yes, I think that's it. And you need to believe that if He doesn't heal you physically then He will still know what He's doing.'

'I need to stop fighting against dying.'

'I think you do.'

244

'I get scared because sometimes I hear God saying about trusting Me even unto death. That must mean I'm going to die.'

'I don't know. Ask God to reveal it to you.'

And so we pray. It is the first time I have prayed for a week. I ask God's forgiveness for relying on alcohol and for turning away from Him. I ask too that He helps me accept the plan He has for me, whatever it is. I cry a lot and pour out my heart to God about how angry and let-down and discouraged I feel. After I have finished, Ellie tucks me up on the sofa with a cup of tea and puts on a disc of worship songs.

'Rest,' she says. 'Just rest and let your mind be quiet.'

I feel very peaceful and very loved. The struggle and the fight have gone and I feel the safety of knowing that I am still God's child. He loves me and cares for me and I have to trust Him. I sleep.

I dream and see an old man, very old; his skin is wrinkled and he is dressed like a Hebrew. He walks up the mountain slowly and he is weeping. Behind him walks a young man who is strong and there is a spring in his step. He carries a bunch of sticks on his back. 'Father, we are almost there.' I realize it is Abraham and his son Isaac. Now I see why the old man is weeping. He must sacrifice his only son, on whom his line depends. With the sticks Isaac builds an altar. 'We have no sacrifice,' he says. 'God will provide,' replies his father. Then he places Isaac, his only son, on the altar and takes out his knife. I see the shiny blade catch the sun as Abraham raises it high above his head and begins to weep again. The beads of sweat soak his brow with sorrow as he contemplates what he must do. As he is about to plunge the sword, a figure appears, white-clothed and tall, just like the Presence. 'Stop!' yells the angel and grabs the knife from the old man's hand in the nick of time. 'Phew! That was a close thing,' laughs Isaac and gets up from the altar. The dream has a clear message but I'm not sure I want to believe it in case my hopes are dashed again.

The following day, 5 October, I pray: 'Lord, I could do with some encouragement today.'

A little later the phone rings. It is Mr Grimer.

'Mary, I've been looking at all your scans today. It is very strange.'

'Why?'

'Well, your latest scan shows that this tumour thing – well, I'm not sure how to put it, but it is smaller than on the previous scan.'

Silence.

'Oh!'

245

'We need to repeat some tests. Can you come up for a bone scan in three weeks? On 27 October?'

'Sure. Yes, of course.'

'I really don't know what is going on here.'

'No, neither do I.' I put down the phone.

'Yes! Yes! Yes! Thank you, God! Wow! That was some encouragement!' I put on one of my worship discs and sing at the top of my voice. 'Yes! Yes! Come on! God, come on! I know You can heal me, I just know it!'

I tell Richard and Ellie about the scan result, but nobody else.

'Maybe this tumour is going to be shrunk and then it will respond to chemotherapy treatment.'

'Maybe God is healing you miraculously,' adds Ellie. I look at her curiously. 'Well, it's possible,' she adds lamely.

'Not probable. But yes – it is possible.'

'We need to visit the Elders again. Tell them the score and pray for total healing,' she says. 'You know me – I'm a nurse, feet on the ground, good old common sense, but this is what we have been asking for. We have to believe it possible.'

Wednesday 6 October. I hardly dare say it. Today I have not had any symptoms from my tumour. It is the first day in six months when I have not had to dry my hair or change my clothes because of the sweats. It might be a one-off. Let's wait and see. I'm not getting my hopes up …

Saturday 9 October. Three days now – no sweats, no wheezing and I'm feeling stronger. I've changed my Fentanyl patch from the highest dose to medium-strength. I'll see what happens to the pain. My breasts are back to normal too – no milk at all.

Sunday 10 October. The pain is less. It is definitely getting less. I record all my medication and I have not needed any painkillers apart from the patch for the last two days. Normally I take about twelve puffs of my inhaler, and now the dose is right down. I'm swopping my Fentanyl patch for the smallest dose to see if I get pain. Today I changed Bethany's nappy for the first time in months.

Sunday 17 October. I am now on the smallest Fentanyl patch. I have been reducing the tablets I take for the poison symptoms because I have not had any sweats or an asthma attack for ten days. I am getting stronger. I am definitely getting stronger. I can walk up the stairs more easily. I can lift up my darling Bethany again. I look healthier, I know I do. Today, at church, somebody told me how much better I look. Something else happened, too: I had some prophecies. Two members of the church came up to me; neither could have had any idea about the scan. They both said that God had told them I was being healed. Awesome, totally awesome. I was so encouraged and I asked them to carry on praying. Could it be? Could it really be that I am getting better after all the long days of illness? I have to stay sensible. It might just be a time of improvement although I cannot imagine why. I could not bear my hopes to be dashed again.

Monday 18 October. Today I went to worship group practice. I have not been able to sing with them since my thoracotomy. It was amazing to see their faces when I walked into church. We had a fantastic time praising God and then at the end we all prayed some more for my healing. I have now stopped all my medication, apart from the smallest Fentanyl patches. Still no poison symptoms! I can't believe I am not taking all those tablets. I feel so brilliant. I am so much stronger and my fingers are not as fat as they were!

Thursday 21 October. Today I cooked a meal for Richard. It was only pasta but he said it was the best meal I ever made. It is eight months since I did that. Can you believe I burnt the garlic bread? We still ate it! No pain and no symptoms. Something is definitely happening.

Friday 22 October. Today Alison phoned from Swansea. A member of their church had another prophecy for me. It was a verse of scripture from John's gospel: 'This sickness shall not end in death.' That's what the verse says, I checked it. I can hardly dare to hope she is right. I can hardly dare thank God just in case it doesn't happen. It is so exciting and yet so frightening. What if the scan shows no change? Maybe this is all my imagination. But how can it be? I've stopped all my medication and now I am symptom-free. I am on a quarter of the Fentanyl dose I was on three weeks ago and I have no pain, none at all. Please, God, please let it be true. Please let me get well. I keep looking at myself in the mirror and asking if it is true, and all I see is a reflection of a woman I have not seen for many months. I think it might be true. I really do. But I cannot say it yet. I need to see the scan first.

Tuesday 26 October. Surreal. I spent the day with Ceri and we went to the hospice clinic. I almost cancelled my appointment but then I changed my mind at the last minute. Something told me I should go and yet I did not feel scared. Ceri came into the doctor's room with me. I talked about death row. But, you know, I'm kind of wondering if maybe – just maybe – I might escape. Maybe this is a last-minute reprieve. This evening I was anointed again by the Elders. They know the scan is tomorrow. I am beginning to feel very nervous. I am so excited at my improvement but if the scan shows a problem … how will I feel? The Elders prayed for me to accept the results, whatever. Afterwards Ceri and I had a chat and I felt I needed to put everything right in my life – to be completely free of anything on my conscience. I wrote a letter to a friend: we had a bad argument, so I wrote saying sorry and posted it.

Then Ceri said a strange thing. 'I've been thinking about the story of Abraham,' she said. 'It keeps coming into my mind. I just thought I should remind you that God intervened right at the last moment when death was staring Isaac in the face. Does that mean anything to you?' Did it? You bet! I know I shall not sleep a wink tonight.

Wednesday 27 October. Today is the day – bone scan repeat. Today I will find out how big the Blob is. I think it will be smaller, I really do. I am so much better. My symptoms have gone completely. For three weeks now I have got through every day with no poison effects. My pain has resolved, too – I am still on the smallest dose of Fentanyl but I haven't needed anything else at all for breakthrough pain. I am stronger. I look healthy again. In fact, I look great. A lot of people have noticed I am looking well. I can put on my make-up and style my hair unaided. I can cook and shop and look after the children. My asthma has stopped and I only use the inhaler before I go swimming – and I have been swimming! I can wear my original wedding ring and my eyes are no longer swollen. Instead of being crippled with pain, I can move freely again.

Ellie picks me up from home and we drive to Birmingham. I suppose we are both desperately hoping it will be good news but we do not want to get our hopes up. First we go to the isotope department and I receive an injection of radioactive material. I remember the very first time Mr Peach explained the test to me.

We have to wait four hours before I can return to have pictures of my body taken. Normally I am anxious and tense, but Ellie and I just laugh and laugh. We eat a huge plateful of tortillas and talk about the times we have shared. The hours fly and at last Ellie checks her watch. 'Okay – time to go. The scan is due in fifteen minutes.'

I lie down on the scanner and wait for my pictures to develop. Ellie is in the next room but can hear everything. It is difficult to see the pictures this time but I strain and strain until I catch a glimpse.

No Blob! I cannot see a Blob!

'I want to take a special view,' says the radiographer, 'just to be sure.'

'Is there a problem?' I ask.

'No, but I need to make sure I have the best pictures,' he answers.

I sit on the scanner, more than a little embarrassed, with my bottom directly over the camera. I have to admit I feel a little exposed.

The radiographer suddenly asks me a question.

'Can I just check your details?'

'Sure.'

I answer his queries – name, address, date of birth. My bottom is still firmly applied to the camera. But I don't care. I know he is surprised, and that must mean good news.

He adds, apologetically: 'It's just … the form says you have a bone secondary and I'm not seeing anything on the scan.'

'Right.'

'Both views are clear. I don't understand it.'

Inside I am singing 'Halleluia! Halleluia!' I wonder what Ellie is thinking.

'I don't understand it, either,' I say and hear my friend coughing loudly in the waiting room.

'Well, you may as well get dressed,' he adds, bewildered. 'The doctors need to see these. You haven't had any treatment, have you?'

'No,' I laugh, 'no treatment.'

'Just prayer,' adds Ellie, as she hands me my clothes.

'Come on, quick, let's find a window,' I say, dragging my friend.

'Why?'

'I want to look at these films, that's why.'

'Naughty doctor!'

'I don't care. I have to see them!'

My heart is racing and I feel flushed with total and utter joy.

Because I know, you see, being a doctor, that if the radiographer can't see it, it isn't there.

I shall never forget the window. It has little wire squares running through it, a little like the books we used in junior school for doing sums.

I hold the pictures to the light and scrutinize them. I see the outline of my bones. There are no differences between the two halves of my pelvis. There are no Blobs.

I stare harder again.

'I can't see anything sinister, Ellie. Can you?'

'Nope, but I'm no expert.'

'Ellie, I truly think it's clear, I do!'

'Come on then, let's get back to clinic. We need to know!'

We hand in the scan. The waiting room is gloomy and depressing. The paint on the wall is lime green and peeling. The atmosphere is cluttered and claustrophobic. We wait. The minutes tick by.

'They are being a long time, Ellie,' I say.

'Come on, chill out. It's going to be fine. I just know.'

'So what do I say, O Wise One, if the scan is clear? Do I tell them what we really believe? Am I brave enough?'

'Listen, I haven't gone through 3 a.m. phone calls for nothing. Don't sit on the fence – say how it is.'

The door opens. Mr Grimer walks in, followed by Dr Spooner.

I shall never forget. He sits on the coffee table. He looks at me with incredulous incomprehension. 'Mary!' He is shaking his head. 'Have you seen these scans?'

I'm a doctor, for goodness sake! Of course I've seen these scans! But am I going to admit it? I don't think so!

'Mmmm,' I say, 'I had a quick peek.'

'You look great!' says Dr Spooner.

'Well, I feel really well. I have no symptoms and my pain has gone.'

'What about your medication?' asks Mr Grimer.

'I've stopped it. I don't need it. My pain has gone, my symptoms are gone. I feel better. I can pick Bethany up. I'm not weak any more. And I'm weaning myself off the Fentanyl.'

'You are a new woman,' says Mr Grimer, smiling. 'Not what we would expect from a terminally ill patient. You're bouncy and bubbly and you look fantastic – totally different.'

'And the scans?' I ask.

'Clear. Completely clear!'

The third miracle.

Thank you, God.

He continues: 'We do not have a medical explanation for what has happened. None whatsoever.'

'Are you sure you couldn't have been mistaken? I mean, have you discussed other diagnoses?'

'Yes,' says Mr Grimer. 'We've considered them all but nothing fits. You have a bone secondary and you are dying. We do nothing to you. You get better. You are in a category of your own – completely inexplicable!'

I shall not die but I shall live.

Ellie and I exchange huge grins and I know I would not have made it without her.

'Do you have any other explanation?' asks Mr Grimer, 'because we really don't.'

'Go on,' say Ellie's eyes. 'Tell it!'

'Well,' I say, tentatively. 'I'm a Christian. We've all been praying. I believe God can heal people.'

I look to my friend for encouragement.

'The only explanation I have,' I continue, hesitantly, unsure of being laughed out of the room, 'is that this is a miracle.'

A short, expectant pause. I look into the eyes of an expert.

'Yes,' he answers. 'I'll buy that.'

Epilogue

The hospice clinic is depressingly familiar. Even the tatty, well-thumbed magazines have not changed. The faces have, though. I am surrounded by a new group of frightened patients. They wait quietly, nervously, sadly, contemplating the silent, deadly advance of mutinous cells. It is February 2000 and I am sitting, hiding, behind the refuge of an out-dated article – 'Countdown to the Millennium'. I smile as I recall the lead-up to our own family celebration which took place in the euphoric aftermath of the third miracle ...

I returned to work as a psychiatrist in December 1999. Only ten months earlier, in February of the same year, I packed away my stetho-scope, fearing even to look at it and contemplate the loss of the medical vocation I love so much. Once again I am working as a physician, caught up in the desire to heal and help. After twelve years of post-graduate training, Richard has secured a post as Consultant in Anaesthesia and Intensive Care Medicine at the Princess of Wales Hospital, Bridgend – the same job for which he was interviewed when I was so ill, the previous July. He and I are settled for the foreseeable future and we do have a future now. At last our family has some stabil-ity. Time is still running for our love. Together. O God, thank you we are together. Let nothing put us asunder. All you need is love, and a cure, and time.

I never thought I would see the third millennium. As I packed up the basket laden with rugs, torches and blankets, champagne and choco-lates on 31 December 1999, my heart sang. Adam, now seven, and Bethany, almost two, sat side by side on the sofa watching worldwide events. Being with my children, thinking about the future without the death sentence hanging over me, was celebration enough for a whole lifetime. I could not help but look back to that first New Year's Eve lived in the shadow of the Limpet, 31 December 1982, when my life changed. That was the night I first prayed for three miracles. How confused and disappointed I was as a seventeen-year-old, trying to make sense of God's purposes. Now, in the last hour of the second millennium, things seemed very different. My unlooked-for first and second miracles – my children – laughed and giggled as they welcomed in a new era.

I shook my head as once again I experienced the utter relief, the total joy, of the third miracle. I remembered, as a seventeen-year-old, asking God for it. Now, seventeen years on, He had granted it. 'I'm clear! I'm not dying! I'm alive!' I said out loud to convince myself of the certain and glorious truth. Richard entered the kitchen whistling 'Auld Lang Syne'.

'What are you muttering about?' he joked.

'Tell me it's true. I'm not dreaming, am I?'

'It's true, Mary. You're better – completely.' He gave me a massive hug. 'You've been healed. Your scans are clear. You're not dying. And if you don't get a move on, we're going to miss the arrival of the twenty-first century.'

'It's incredible. Amazing. Awesome. Miraculous.' I smiled up at Richard and he ruffled my hair.

'It is. Sometimes I can't take it in, either.'

We all headed out into the dark, cold night to the Wenallt Hill. It was brightly lit with bonfires. Hundreds of revellers were gathered, singing and enjoying themselves. Hard to believe this was the place where I planned a funeral and picked out a burial plot. As the countdown started to 1 January 2000, Richard and I encircled our two children tightly in our arms. Fireworks exploded in a dozen different colours as the champagne overflowed and we kissed ecstatically …

Dr Jefferson arrives in clinic, a bundle of case-notes tucked under her arm. She waves me into her office.

'Mary, you look great,' she greets me. 'Is the sparkle real or artificial?'

'Very definitely real!' I reply, smiling.

'So fill me in then. Tell me what has been happening.'

'Where do I start?'

'Start with the miracle, when your scan result was clear – back in October, was it?'

'It was 27 October. The date is forever etched in my memory.'

'What was it like? How did you feel, going from seeing me here one day to being told your scan was clear the next?'

'I felt ...' I search for the words because I have still not found any which can adequately describe it, '... I felt totally and completely euphoric. It was like a taste of heaven, I guess. It was sheer, brilliant joy dripping into every part of my soul. It was like touching another realm, magnificent, divine. I was – am – so full of enormous energy. I feel reborn. Nothing can ever be normal or boring or ordinary again.'

There is a silence as Melanie takes in what I have said.

'Now I am totally drug and symptom-free. No pain, back to my normal activities, looking after the kids, working, swimming – all the usual stuff I used to do before the relapse. I feel completely well again.'

'And your check-ups? Are you still clear?'

'Yes. I had my first check-up recently at the Royal Orthopaedic Hospital in Birmingham. My tests are normal. My case has been discussed all over the world now. The oncologists are still trying to come up with an answer but there isn't a medical explanation that fits.'

'Well, you know the answer, don't you?'

'Yes, I do. I know something happened to me beyond human understanding. Something divine. A miracle.'

'What about the sceptics? There must be people who don't believe it was a miracle. Does that bother you?'

'Well, I guess some people have questioned whether it was God who healed me ... and let's face it, nobody can prove the existence of God. But they still admit there is no reasonable explanation for what has happened to me. A lot of doctors would call it "spontaneous remission". I call it a miracle. But either way it doesn't really matter. It is still a story of hope.'

'What do you mean?'

'To some, it shows the way faith can sustain and the amazing love of a mighty God intervening. To others, it demonstrates a way to cope – the ability to see their own situation positively, however desperate it may be. And it shows, too, the indomitable power of the human spirit to overcome and to conquer.'

'So how did all the publicity come about? I couldn't believe it when I saw you on the front page of the *Mirror* back in December.'

We laugh together as I recount another incredible series of events.

'It was like this. After I had seen the doctors in Birmingham, I knew I should tell the story. I just knew it. I had to turn my experience into something positive. So, when I returned home from Birmingham, I wrote down what had happened over the previous few months since

254

being diagnosed as terminal. I couldn't get the words down fast enough. The energy and the euphoria just translated themselves into writing and I came up with the booklet I sent you.'

'Yes, it's in your notes here,' replies Melanie, pulling out my ten-page booklet telling the story of the miracle.

'I distributed the booklet through local churches, and the story was picked up by a Christian journalist, Rob James, who wrote an article for a Christian newspaper. It inspired a lot of people and made it on to the front page, so then he contacted the *Mirror* to see if they wanted to cover it.'

'And they did?'

'Yes, I told my story to one of their journalists, Rod Chaytor, who confirmed it with Mr Grimer, my specialist in Birmingham. He told the *Mirror* that Cardiff had phoned him in desperation, saying: "Can you do anything to save this woman's life?" Mr Grimer said my symptoms were "wholly and indisputably genuine" and my case was "unique". He also said that if it wasn't a metastasis in my pelvis from my original sarcoma then he didn't know what it was, and a disappearing metastasis was indeed a miracle. It ended up on the front page of all editions – massive picture, "miracle" headline and a two-page spread inside. The full treatment!'

'I think the hospital shop ran out of copies by about ten o' clock,' jokes Melanie. 'Everybody was talking about it.'

'Well, after that it just went completely crazy. The phone didn't stop ringing. The story was covered on the radio, television, the Internet – it went worldwide. God certainly wanted people to hear about it.'

'And what next? A book?'

'Yes. We're on chapter four.' I beam at Melanie and she smiles back.

'So what do you want to do now about this clinic?'

'I guess I need to draw a line. Move on. I'm healed for now. And it's strange, but the fear I always felt – living with the sword above my head – has gone now. I'm no longer frightened of the cancer. That is part of the healing, too. So could you discharge me?' I add.

Melanie leans back in her chair. 'I've never been part of a miracle before,' she says. 'Sometimes I've seen people whose symptoms have improved dramatically with prayer … But a genuine healing – this is the first time.'

'So …?'

'Off you go. Discharged. But keep in touch!'

I walk across the room, my heart pounding with joy.

'And send me a copy of the book!'

'I promise!'

I walk down the long corridor and out of the hospital towards the garden where I saw the vision of the valley. As I walk away I bid a final farewell. I am not saying goodbye to the cancer, for who knows whether I shall remain well? No, I am saying goodbye to the fear. I have looked my enemies in the face now. The Limpet, the Penny and the Blob. They were ugly and cruel and brought me so much pain. But the fear was worst of all. And I have survived and conquered the fear. It has been defeated by a perfect and divine Love.

Later that day I approach the door of an empty house with a set of keys in my hand. This is our new home in Cardiff. We have given it a Welsh name, 'Gwyrthfan', meaning 'place of miracles'. Adam and Bethany push past me, excitedly looking for their new bedrooms. I hear their voices echoing through the empty rooms.

Bethany runs up to me and flings her arms around my legs. 'Mummy! Mummy!' she yells enthusiastically. She knows and recognizes me as Mummy now. I am watching my tiny daughter grow up. Her future is no longer apart from mine. She can now use a spoon and feed herself. I have bought her first potty! I have put her name down for a place at the local nursery and I shall be able to take her there myself. She has brought home her first messy two-year-old's painting. I have watched her play piggy-back with Adam and I shall watch them become best friends. So many things we take for granted … More milestones await me. I shall help her hang out her first Christmas stocking and build her first snowman. I shall see her perform as an angel in her first nativity. Maybe I shall dress her in her uniform for her first day at school. Perhaps I shall teach her about make-up and clothes, her periods and boys. Girl things. Exams and wedding dresses. She will know me as warmth and friendship. So much to hope for. So much to live for. So much I thought I would miss out on. And now … now she will remember me.

My life again seems full of new beginnings. How glibly we say those words. New … life … beginnings. If I could go back and change things, would I? When I think of the prayer so innocently said, 'Use me, Father, for Your service', would I choose different words? Would I ask for perfect health and long life? No! For I have caught sight of eternity. I have glimpsed beyond the grave. I have seen a vision of something more powerful than anything we frail mortals can comprehend. Something that makes us appear ridiculous and insignificant in our strivings for answers and solutions, like grasshoppers jumping from place to place and hope to hope but finding nothing of consequence. For I know a God who meets me in my pain and longings, in my joy and my despair. I know a God who became mortal, a God who died and a God who conquered death. I have a certain hope and a glorious future. I know a God whose name is Love.

> *I didn't die. I lived!*
> *And now I'm telling the world what God has done.*
> *God tested me, He pushed me hard,*
> *But He didn't hand me over to Death.*
> *Amen.*

Dr Mary Self
Cardiff
27 October 2000

Acknowledgements

Richard ... for better, for worse, for richer, for poorer, in sickness and in health. Our love is my inspiration.

Adam and Bethany Lydia, whose smiles, cuddles and laughter have made it all worth it ... I survived for you.

I have always been blessed with the unconditional and unfailing love of my family; Mum, Dad, Martin, Franny, Hellie and Adrian. You developed and nurtured my will to live. Thankyou for being a part of my story and for allowing me to tell it.

There are literally hundreds of medical, nursing and paramedical staff who have been involved in my care over the last seventeen years. It is impossible to name them all. Their dedication and compassion has been unfailing. There are many whose care has been beyond the call of duty. I am alive because of their skills.

Mr Barry Peach, Orthopaedic Surgeon, Victoria Hospital, Blackpool.
Mr John Jackett, Prosthetist, Royal Preston Hospital, Preston.
Dr N. K. Gupta, Oncologist, Christie Hospital, Manchester.
Mrs Sue Hancock, Counsellor, Swansea Christian Resource Centre,
    Swansea.
Mr Nigel Davies, Obstetrician, University Hospital Wales, Cardiff.
Mrs Ruth Nash, Perinatal Bereavement Counsellor, Llandough
    Hospital, Cardiff.
Dr Melanie Jefferson, Palliative Care Consultant, Cardiff.
Dr Siôn Edwards, General Practitioner, Cardiff.
Mr Robert Grimer, Orthopaedic Surgeon, Birmingham.

Rod, thankyou is not enough. Your loyal support and friendship have enabled me to write my story. We have cried and laughed a lot in travelling this journey together. I could not have returned to the dark days of fear and despair alone. This book would not have been written without your vision and inspiration. Love always.

I owe a huge debt of gratitude and probably a dozen crates of champagne to my 'Merry Men & Women'. You helped me find strength, dignity and laughter in the Valley of the Shadow of Death. Ellie – best friend a girl could have, survivingly yours …

Rod and I wish to thank Jeff Braham, of Coventry University, for his appraisal of our efforts and for proofreading the final typescript.